DATE DUE

JUN 2 8 1995	
FEB 1 8 2002	3598/07

PHILOSOPHY, RELIGION AND PSYCHOTHERAPY

Essays in the Philosophical Foundations of Psychotherapy

Edited by

Paul W. Sharkey
University of Southern Mississippi

UNIVERSITY
PRESS OF
AMERICA

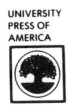

Library of Congress Catalog Card Number: 81-40828

FOR

ALL THOSE WHOSE VOCATION
IS THE WELL BEING OF MAN

"Know then thyself, presume not God
to scan;
The proper study of mankind is man."

Alexander Pope

ACKNOWLEDGEMENTS

Major credit for this volume must go to its contributors without whose patient cooperation it would not have been possible. Therefore, to Professors Friedman, Macklin, Needleman, Scott and Sullivan for sharing their philosophical expertise and to Professors Morris, Rychlak, Sollod, Szasz and Weiskopf-Joelson for sharing their insights and experiences in psychotherapy, a very special thanks.

The idea for this volume began three years ago through conversations with graduate students interested in the philosophical presuppositions of psychotherapeutic models. A special thanks to Charles Gambrell, one of those students, who was particularly helpful in researching the literature relating to this issue. It was from the list of authors of those works that the invitation and selection of contributions to this volume was drawn.

Several typists aided in the preparation of manuscripts, most notably Linda Gambrell whose excellent skills were very much appreciated in re-typing edited manuscripts early in the project and to Normia Washington who prepared the final typescript for the volume. There are no doubt still some typographical errors which may be found in the volume for which I take full responsibility. But I owe a debt of gratitude to those who helped me proofread the typescript without whose assistance there would have been even more.

To my chairman, Dr. Forrest Wood, who patiently listened to my expressions of frustrations during the period of this project and finally, to my wife Karen, a student of both psychology and philosophy whose reassurance and advise, not only as a wife, but also as a student of psychology is deeply appreciated.

CONTRIBUTING AUTHORS

Maurice Friedman (Philosophy)
San Diego State University

Ruth Macklin (Philosophy)
Albert Einstein College of Medicine

Joseph E. Morris (Psychology)
Timber Hills Mental Health Services

Jacob Needleman (Philosophy)
San Francisco State University

Joseph F. Rychlak (Psychology)
Purdue University

Charles E. Scott (Philosophy)
Vanderbuilt University

Robert N. Sollod (Psychology)
Cleveland State University

Roger J. Sullivan (Philosophy)
University of South Carolina

Thomas Szsaz (Psychiatry)
State University of New York, Syracuse

Edith Weisskopf-Joelson (Psychology)
University of Georgia

CONTENTS

PREFACE

PSYCHOTHERAPY AND THE PHILOSOPHY OF HEALTH CARE

Recent history has seen the rise of considerable interest in issues broadly characterized under the heading of values in health care. Questions about abortion, euthanasia and genetics seem to appear daily in the popular press and such specialities as bioethics and philosophy of medicine have emerged on the academic scene in response to a perceived crisis in the conceptual and ethical foundations of biomedical health care practices.

Symptomatic of our age however, the emphasis in this concern to find sound values upon which to base the healing arts has been limited primarily to those arts which have as their object the health of the body with little or no attention being payed to those which are concerned with "healing the mind." This in itself says something about the kinds of values about which we are most concerned. Yet, the implications of practicing an "art of healing the mind" which is without sound ethical and conceptual foundations are at least if not more dangerous than for those involved in healing the body. If there is to be a coherent and comprehensive view of health and health care, then mental health and those who purport to be engaged in the healing of the mind must not be excluded from the same kind of reevaluation that the biomedical health care professions are presently undergoing. With a view toward that end, the purpose of this volume is to begin the task of investigating some of the more basic ethical and conceptual principles involved in psychotherapy--the art of healing the mind.

Since the primary goal of this work is to stimulate interdisciplinary research in the foundations of psychotherapy, as already begun in the biomedical health care fields, it was thought that it would be appropriate for it to be composed of contributions from professionals representing the various disciplines directly concerned with the values and concepts inherent in psychotherapeutic practices rather than by a single author. Thus, though perhaps somewhat different in style and approach owing to their respective disciplines, the essays in this collection have been chosen and organized around a central theme concerned with a common set of issues.

The first section consists of four essays which

address themselves to some of the more basic concepts and presuppositions of psychotherapeutic practices. Beginning with an analysis of the ethical presuppositions and potential conflicts inherent in any psychotherapeutic model, the first essay argues that a completely value neutral psychotherapy is impossible and that given this fact what is needed is an open, honest and responsible recognition of the value presuppositions of psychotherapies and their practicioners. The second essay attempts to address itself to precisely this demand by explicating the more fundamental presuppositions of therapies based on humanistic psychology while the third essay addresses itself to the issue of the "scientific" and "non-scientific" aspects of psychotherapy and similarities of psychotherapy to religious and educational models. The last paper of this section raises the question of whether or not either of the so-called "humanistic" or "scientific" based therapies are adequate in their philosophical images of man and his relation to the wholeness of being, calling for a radical reconsideration of these issues as they relate to contemporary psychotherapy.

The essays of the second section represent initial attempts to deal with some of the more basic questions raised in the first section. Thus, the first paper of this section concerns itself with the concept of the "wholeness of being" as it relates to the practice of psychotherapy while the second essay is devoted to an analysis of the "image of man" in the same regard. The third essay investigates the relation between philosophical, religious and scientific aspects of the origins of psychotherapy in Freudian psychoanalysis with the last essay of the section being devoted to an analysis of the philosophical aspects of five kinds of contemporary psychotherapeutic models.

One of the central and most persistent themes which emerges from these essays is that of the relation of psychotherapy to religion. This theme constitutes the final section of our study. The first paper raises in general the question of the status of psychotherapy vis a vis religion and its potential for political and social abuse. The second essay addresses itself to values and concepts held in common by the western religious tradition and humanistic psychology, suggesting the possibility of a reconcilliation between contemporary psychology and religion. The third essay, on the other hand, argues that such a reconcilliation is not possible without major revision of at least one fundamental issue of conflict between contemporary humanistic psycho-therapy and traditional western religion. Completing this section and the collection as a whole is an essay written by a therapist and scholar whose personal and professional experiences are uniquely well suited to address the issue to the "therapeutic" aspects of re-ligious and political philosophies.

Though some of the essays of this collection a-ttempt to offer initial suggestions for answering some of the questions raised, the major intent of this volume is to provoke questioning--it is intended to provoke re-consideration of the presuppositions of psychotherapy and "mental health." If the reader sometimes feels that like Kierekgaard our purpose "is to create difficulties everywhere," then know that it is done in the belief that like life, "the unexamined therapy is not worth practicing."

BASIC CONCEPTS AND PRESUPPOSITIONS

BASIC CONCEPTS AND PRESUPPOSITIONS

For over two centuries the authority of science
has reigned supreme in defining matters of truth and
reality. It is not even a small exageration to say
that the very nature and existence of contemporary
society rests upon the foundation of the achievements
of modern science.

While it would be foolish to deny the value of
the insights and achievements brought by modern science, it would be equally foolhardy to ignore the problems which have resulted from modern man's scientific
obsession. In today's world, being respectable is almost synonymous with being "scientific." But not
everything which calls itself science really is and
even within genuine science the tendency to separate
the world of "facts" from the world of values has lead
many to adopt the illusion of science as "objective"
and "value neutral."

The fact of the matter is, however, that not even
genuine or "pure" science is completely value neutral,
still less those disciplines which for professional
acceptance and prestige have proclaimed themselves to
be "sciences" in the hope of hiding behind the charade
of this objective value neutrality. Nowhere is recognition of this more important than in those disciplines concerned with health and health care. The very
concept of health is itself at once both descriptive
and normative. "Health" is first and formost a value
concept. The apparently descriptive question: What
is it to be healthy? presupposes the more fundamentally normative question of what should a "healthy"
person be able to do?

The problem of defining health is difficult
enough in the biomedical health care professions where,
at least to some extent, minimal physiological criteria
can be employed to set boundaries in defining conflicts
of values. The situation in the mental health field,
however, is complicated not only by the same kind of
problems which face biomedical health care practitioners but also by those which come from the general lack
of reasonably uniform and professionally agreed upon
therapeutic procedures for the treatment of "mental
illness." The situation in psychotherapy may be described by analogy in the biomedical field as being
somewhat akin to the conflict between chiropractic

3

and traditional medical therapies but complicated many fold due to the proliferation and diversity of therapeutic philosophies which include themselves under the umbrella of "psychotherapy." Each of these therapeutic philosophies presuppose and promote, whether realized or not, a particular set of values. These values can and sometimes do conflict not only with those of other therapeutic philosophies but also with the values of those by whom and upon whom the therapy is applied.

As the first essay of this section argues, a completely value free therapy is impossible, as are the conflicts of values which naturally arise as the result of the differing value perspectives of the therapeutic model, therapist and client. What is needed is not an attempt to rid therapies of their value content but rather a conscientious and systematic effort to make their value presuppositions clearly manifest. Only then will we be in a position to be able to judge intelligently the axiological merits of a psychotherapeutic philosophy.

One psychotherapeutic philosophy, or rather school of such philosophies, which has shown some sensitivity to questions of value even to the point of confessing its own values and conceptual presuppositions is "humanistic" psychotherapy. Stressing "self actualization" to a high degree, humanistic therapies tend to see themselves as more person oriented than therapies which have emerged solely from the experimental-behaviorist mentality of "scientific" psychotherapies. Such humanistic therapies have a basically phenomenological view of method and epistemology combined with an existentialist's view of human nature. In other words, humanistic psychotherapies represent the practical application of the philosophical world view of phenomenology and existentialism in the form of "therapy." Thus, when one enters into such therapy his "cure" will consist not only of the mere alleviation of his distress but also in his acceptance of or conversion to the world view and view of the self which that therapy presupposes.

Sensitive to this issue, the second essay of this section focuses on those concepts and presuppositions which are considered basic to the world view of humanistic psychotherapy. Since no therapy can be completely value free or presuppositionless the

4

recognition that humanistic psychotherapy is really a
kind of applied philosophy is in-itself no criticism
of its validity. On the contrary, it signifies a step
in the direction of the kind of self reflective and
responsible philosophical honesty with which all
therapeutic philosophies should be evaluated.

The fact that in many cases being "cured" under
a given therapeutic model means adopting or being converted to the world view upon which it is based raises
some fundamental questions regarding the nature of the
therapeutic enterprise itself. Whether it claims to
be scientific, humanistic or even supernatural makes
no difference. What is at issue here is the kind of
activity therapy represents regardless of its claims
concerning its theoretical underpinnings. As our third
essay argues, when one looks at the <u>activity</u> of therapy
it may seem to resemble religion more than science.
Often the "client" is progressively persuaded toward
adopting a "correct" view of himself and his relation
to the world through certain ritualistic practices
which are to be adhered to religiously if a "cure" is
to be forthcoming. Much like the disciplines of
mystical religions, psychotherapies attempt to lead
their disciples ever closer to that state of enlightenment in which their suffering will be overcome and
their true selves realized. Upon "being cured" they
may even report a "conversion experience" as personally profound and meaningful as those claimed for
religion.

Though there may be some similarity between the
enterprise of psychotherapy and religious disciplines
this does not necessarily imply that psychotherapy is
merely disguised religion. Instead, the fact that
both religion and psychotherapy may be engaged in similar activities, though often from widely differing
perspectives, points to a more basic characteristic of
the practices of both. Both religion and psychotherapy
are engaged in the enterprise of attempting to guide
their followers to the recognition of what, according
to each, is in the best interests of the "client" or
disciple. Seen in this way the kind of activity represented by psychotherapy is neither science nor religion but rather education. And, it is education in
its most basic philosophic sense--the quest to "know
thyself."

From a purely philosophical perspective the very

5

existence of a need for psychotherapy could itself be viewed as a symptom of a more basic underlying problem--the problem of our failure, both individually and collectively, to heed the philosophical imperative "know thyself!" Just as in the biomedical health care fields, if we are not careful to distinguish symptoms from causes we may be seduced into believing that our therapies are curative when in fact they may only be cosmetic. Also just as in biomedical treatments the success of palliative therapies which effectively eliminate the distress of our symptoms may in the end be more dangerous than the conditions for which they were designed by anesthetizing us from their root cause.

The fundamental question that is at issue is the nature of man. Psychotherapy cannot responsibly be conducted independent of philosophy and anthropology for the problem man faces is the discovery of his own nature and its (his) relation to the fullness of Being. As our last essay of this section argues, the history of any enterprise which fails to heed this fundamental aspect of the human condition is at best the history of an illusion.

VALUES IN PSYCHOANALYSIS
AND PSYCHOTHERAPY: A
SURVEY AND ANALYSIS*

Ruth Macklin

It is acknowledged by psychiatrists, psychologists, and philosophers alike that the ways in which values enter into the theory and practice of psychotherapy are pervasive and exceedingly complex. The chief aim of this paper will be to explore these varied and complex intersections between values and psychoanalytic and psychotherapeutic concerns, in theory and practice. The analysis presented here will be largely classificatory, for it would seem that such an effort is of crucial necessity for introducing greater clarity and achieving a better understanding of issues that are of considerable importance to individuals and society. Moreover, a clear understanding of the multifarious ways in which values are embedded in psychoanalytic theory and practice is significant both for the further development of psychoanalytic theory and for the implementation of therapeutic practice, policy recommendations, and social reforms.

In addition to its import for professional and lay concerns in the field of psychoanalysis and psychotherapy, this inquiry bears on long-standing philosopical issues in value theory and epistemology--notably, the distinction and intersection between facts and values. Although I shall remain somewhat neutral with respect to traditional and contemporary philosophical positions on the fact-value question, it will emerge in what follows that the distinction is exceedingly difficult to maintain in a rigorous way, both in the explication of psychoanalytic concepts and in the application of those concepts to persons in identifying and treating mental illness. The term 'values' will be used to cover a large and heterogeneous range of notions including the following: preferred goals; actual or ideal norms governing human behavior and therapeutic methodology; prescriptions or directives ('ought' statements) employed by therapists or embodied

---
*Reprinted by permission of the Editor, The American Journal of Psychoanalysis, Vol. 33, No. 2, 1973.

in a psychotherapeutic system; value judgments using the ethical terms 'good', 'bad', 'right', 'wrong', etc., or more general terms with value implications, such as 'successful', 'mature'. 'normal'; ideologies and ethical ideals.

In the remainder of this paper, I shall discuss values in psychoanalysis and psychotherapy as falling into three general categories. The justification for the particular classificatory scheme adopted here is the belief that an analysis along these lines will be fruitful for enabling us to get a closer look, in a systematic way, at the various sorts of value issues embedded in the theory and practice of psychotherapy. The three categories are as follows:

I   Values actually held by the patient or client;

II   Values actually held by the therapist or psychoanalyst;

III   Values implicit or explicit in various psychoanalytic and psychotherapeutic theories.

This way of structuring the issues does not exhaust the value areas pertinent to psychoanalysis and psychotherapy. For example, two further categories that should be borne in mind are: values implicit in the model according to which mental disorders and problems are classified, interpreted, and treated; and value considerations that bear on attempts to define or characterize the basic concepts of mental "health" and mental "illness", "normal" and "abnormal" behavior. Inquiry into these latter areas involves considerations that lie beyond the scope of the present study. (Macklin, 1972, pp 49-70) The classification employed here involves some overlap among the categories, as shown briefly in an example. One of the most pervasive problems in this field is that of identifying particular cases as instances of mental illness. In one study the authors note that different norms of adjustment are employed by different users of the term 'mental illness' and that "usually the use of the phrase 'mental illness' effectively marks the actual norms being applied." (Livermore, 1968, p.80) Moreover, the authors claim that "the usual

reason for variance in diagnosis is a variance in the
theoretical orientation of the diagnosticians."
(Livermore, 1968, p.80) So it is apparent that the
problem of identifying particular cases as instances
of mental illness is affected by different norms adhered to by individual psychiatrists (category II);
by the theoretical orientation to which they subscribe
(category III); and by the particular model according
to which they interpret and explain the psychiatric
disorder. In addition, there are subjective value
biases on the part of psychiatrists that tend to creep
in, further compounding the problem of diagnosis and
identification of mental illness. The above-noted
authors write:

> Probably the most pernicious error is com-
> mited by those who classify as 'sick' be-
> behavior that is aberrant in neither a
> statistical sense nor in terms of any de-
> fensible biological or medical criterion,
> but solely on the bais of the clinician's
> personal ideology of mental health and inter-
> personal relationships. Examples might be
> the current psychiatric stereotype of what a
> good mother or a healthy family must be like,
> or the rejection as 'perverse' of forms of
> sexual behavior that are not biologically
> harmful, are found in many infra-human
> mammals and in diverse human cultures, and
> have a high statistical frequency in our
> own society. (Livermore, 1969, p.79)

What this example serves to show is that there
are a number of different and subtle ways in which
norms and values can affect diagnostic practice--ways
that arise out of personal biases of psychiatrists,
their theoretical orientations, and the values implicit in the very concepts of mental health and mental
illness (e.g., norms of optimum adjustment, well-
functioning, etc.) that are employed in psychiatric
judgments.

Finally, it should be noted that the three categories above proceed from the more particular to the
most general. The first two categories are comprised
of individual persons' (patients' or therapists')
moral beliefs, ethical codes, value judgments, and
behavioral norms; the third category encompasses values

9

at the level of psychoanalytic or psychotherapeutic theory. Of the additional value areas mentioned above, one includes values in psychopathological models, which typically encompass several different theories or theoretical systems. The other additional category deals with the most general notions that enter into all theories, systems and models: the concepts of mental "health" and "illness," "normal" and "abnormal" behavior. No matter what personal moral beliefs and values or methodological norms are adhered to by a psychotherapist, and no matter what values are embodied in various theories or models, they must all come to grips eventually with defining, characterizing, and applying the crucial concepts in this last category. Bearing in mind that each successive category in the classification is likely to encompass problems and issues that arise in the earlier ones, we may now proceed to a discussion of the three value categories.

    I.   Values actually held by the patient or client.

        A.   Moral or ethical codes and precepts believed in or assented to by him.

In this category, we find all those views that are usually held to constitute a person's moral beliefs, whether in the form of a "code of ethics", adherence to a particular moral theory (e.g., egoism, utilitarianism), or a set of ethical generalizations to which a person subscribes. These would include all sorts of views, from affirmation or denial of the Ten Commandments to beliefs that the Protestant Ethic is valuable, capitalism is morally bankrupt, the family should stick together at all costs, abortion is wrong, etc. Here the point is that the rules, codes, or precepts adhered to and acknowledged by the person are general-- they refer not to specific instances, actions, or cases, of a certain type.

        B.   Specific beliefs of the patient or client concerning what he ought to do or what is right for him to do in some particular circumstance.

In this category we find particular ethical judgments under consideration or actually made by a psychiatric patient, e.g., he ought to get divorced, he ought to stop beating his wife, he ought not to engage in extra-marital affairs, he ought to give up his job at the chemical warfare plant, etc. Of course, these sorts of judgments and decisions are paradigmatic of the moral choices and dilemmas faced by all human beings, wheter psychiatric patients or not. But their importance for the psychiatric context rests on two factors. That is, there may be and often is a conflict or gap between what the person generally assents to and what he actually does. Moreover, there may be a conflict between those precepts or rules he claims to assent to generally and what he feels he ought to do in a specific case, which conflict may be attributable to special circumstances, anxiety, neurotic indecision, "acting out" behavior, pervasive weakness of will, conflict between superego and ego, and the like. In the extreme this conflict is characterized as psychological compulsion, as in cases of kleptomania. In the range of neurotic behaviors, a patient finds an inability in such cases of conflict to act in accordance with his acknowledged moral beliefs or value scheme.

The second factor of importance for the psychiatric context lies in the possibility of a divergence between a patient's moral beliefs and similar sorts of beliefs held by a psychoanalyst or therapist. In a work entitled Values in Psychotherapy, Charlotte Buhler emphasized "the fact that basically different value orientations are held by individual patients and therapists alike. There must be room for the consideration of this fact in psychotherapy." (Buhler, 1962, p.16) Thus the different moral beliefs of patient and therapist may affect the actual therapy itself, both in terms of the direction the therapy takes and even the success or failure of the therapy.

The importance of a psychiatric patient's value scheme and commitments is emphasized by a number of writers. Dr. Buhler, in particular, asserts that "it is our conviction that values permeate our development and personality to such a degree that they can never be left out of the picture". (Buhler, 1962, p. X) A factor that Dr. Buhler claims exacerbates this entire problem area in psychotherapy is the vague and shifting value system of contemporary society. (Buhler, 1962, p.6)

Finally, it should be noted that it is often a

11

strong value conflict or indecision about a course of
action in which values are embedded that leads a person initially to seek psychiatric help. In addition,
the success of psychoanalysis or therapy is often
evaluated in terms of the patient's increasing ability
to resolve such conflicts, to act where he was former-
ly incapacitated, and to develop his own value scheme.
As Buhler discusses at length in her book, the extent
to which different therapies actively aid a patient
or client to develop his own value scheme varies greatly from one psychotherapeutic approach to another.
But the salient point that emerges is this. In addition to the more narrowly defined moral beliefs and
precepts noted above under A and B, there are other,
more general value precepts that are crucial to the
understanding and implementation of various psychoanalytic theories and therapies. These more general
precepts embody norms of personal adjustment, well-
being, self-realization, self-actualization, as
characterized and ascribed to by different theories.
More will be said about these below, but it should be
noted here that "successful" therapy (itself a normative notion) is often defined in terms of the degree
to which a patient has internalized some such norms
and precepts, and achieved an adequate self-concept of
happiness, well-being, self-realization, etc., on which
he can act as a well-integrated person. To the extent
that different therapeutic approaches stress different
norms of adjustment, self-realization, and the like,
there remains a possibility and even likelihood of
disagreement among theorists and therapists concerning
the success or failure of therapy and the mental health
or mental illness of a patient, in particular cases.
But it is generally held that whatever specific norms
of adjustment or ideals of well-being are adopted, the
patient himself must develop and be able to act in
accordance with a coherent value scheme, if therapy is
to be counted as a success. (Jahoda, 1958) To this
end, development and realization of what Buhler terms
a patient's "value potential" ("both in terms of the
values he can truly identify with and those he can
bring to materialization") (Buhler, 1968, p.198) comprise a crucial part of psychotherapeutic practice,
and serve as partial criteria employed by therapists
in evaluating the success or failure of psychotherapy
with a particular patient.

II. Values actually held by the therapist

    A. General moral or ethical codes and precepts believed in or assented to by him.

This category is similar to that in IA, except that here the values are those of the therapist. The subjective biases of a clinician may and often do affect his diagnostic practice. Still, in such cases the psychiatrist's judgments are related to the professional concerns of mental health and illness and interpersonal relationships, notwithstanding the fact that such judgments are based on subjective or personal ideology rather than on some consistent objective framework. The parallel situation to that of the patient's moral beliefs and ethical precepts, as discussed in IA, arises in the following way in therapeutic contexts. Often a therapist's own convictions enter the picture and, as Buhler notes, "As far as the therapist's personal standards are concerned, this is an ethical question. The therapist's integrity requires that he maintain his own standards." ("Buhler, 1962, p.199) Buhler cites one case in which a professional gambler came to a therapist with the problem of impotence. The therapist doubted whether his own ethical code allowed him to treat a person who made his living by consciously taking advantage of people. It emerged in this case that the therapist was able to help the patient cope with his specific problem of impotence and also restructure his personality and his life in accordance with ethical values adhered to by the therapist. "The conviction with which (the therapist) continued to work on this case, was justified by his patient's continuous development." (Buhler, 1962, pp. 198-199)

In another case cited by Buhler, one of her own patients subscribed to a value scheme that was inimical to her own. In this connection, Buhler notes that at times "the patient's welfare is endangered by the therapist's taking a stand that is much at variance from the patient's." (Buhler, 1962, pp. 200-201) In the particular case at hand, the patient was a woman for whom it was extremely important that the therapist should be entirely and totally for her. (Buhler, 1962, pp. 201-202) Buhler notes further that the patient wanted the therapist to adopt her own political and religious convictions, rather than that she should be made to identify with the therapist's "silly idealism." Acknowledging that not much could be done in the face of this impasse, Buhler reports that she tried to do what seemed most constructive under the circumstances in continuing therapy with the patient.

There is no clear argument among theorists and therapists on the question of whether or when the therapist should inject his own moral views into the therapeutic process in cases of conflict with those of a patient or indecision about a moral course of action on the part of a patient. (Simkin, 1962, p.209) It is thus apparent that the moral beliefs and general (non-professional) values of the therapist may play an important role in the direction of the therapeutic process and even in its eventual success or failure.

> B. "Professional" ethics: specific beliefs on the part of the analyst or therapist concerning his behavior towards patients in a therapeutic situation

It is important to distinguish this category of values in psychoanalysis and psychotherapy from category III, below. The emphasis here is on values relating to methodological questions and problems faced by the therapist rather than on the values embedded in the theoretical orientation that he espouses. Although this is one area where the categories overlap to some extent and in some cases cannot be separated out for analysis, still the distinction can be maintained by focusing on the methodological aspects here. The point can be made by noting that a set of value questions relating to methodology arises no matter what theoretical position a therapist adopts, and conversely, different value conceptions arise out of alternative psychoanalytic and psychotherapeutic theories even when there is agreement among therapists on the methodological questions. There appear to be three sub-categories in this section.

> (1) Values placed on one or another type of therapeutic methodology by the analyst or therapist

Some of the questions faced by the therapist in this connection are the following: Ought I to tell the patient that what he is doing is right or wrong, good or bad? Ought I to suggest a course of action to a patient that he might follow, or simply help him to find his own? Ought I try to redirect his general value scheme or moral precepts on the grounds that the ones he holds are morally wrong (according to my personal ethical standards) or destructive to him and others (according to my professional judgment)? There is an obvious connection here with issues raised under IIA namely, in those cases where a therapist's own moral views differ from those of the patient. The question here concerns not the therapist's personal values, but rather the norms that are incorporated in his chosen methodology and that might be justified by him on theoretical and/or pragmatic grounds. (Buhler, 1962, p.6)

As already noted, the range of actual positions adopted by different theorists and therapists covers the entire spectrum. Buhler points out, that three historical periods can be distinguished in which a predominant position was held by clinicians. In the first period, Freud himself and some of his earlier pupils speak of "pedagogic measures: that have to be used, "to press the patient into a new decision." This is the "active" approach that has had among its adherents Richard Sterba, Franza Alexander, and S. Ferenczi. In the second period, the psychoanalytic technique is characterized by neutrality, detachment, and non-interference. In the words of Edward Glover, the "abandonment of neutrality" is "the main disadvantage inherent in active methods." (Glover, 1958, p.175) This non-interference approach among psychoanalysts was shared during this period by nonanalytically oriented psychotherapeutic groups, a chief proponent being Carl Rogers, whose "originally 'nondirective' approach (1951) to psychotherapy was prompted by his concern that the patient should remain autonomous in his development and direction." (Buhler, 1962, p.7) In the third period (at present) Buhler notes a return to more active and participating procedures on the part of analysts and therapists, including Rogers himself. (Buhler, 1962, p.8)

Unfortunately, space does not permit a detailed discussion of the contentions of psychoanalysts and

15

psychotherapists in support of these considerations, only a few will be noted briefly here.

(a) In reference to the unnaturalness of the "analyst's anonymity," some writers point out that

> the analyst who feels strongly motivated by social values cannot turn aside from such activities without undermining his own integrity and feelings of self-esteem and any such denial might well affect his relationships with his patients, certainly as much and more so than mere compliance with a technical rule. (Ginsberg, (Buhler), 1962, p.8)

Here the intertwining of two aspects of the value problem--the therapist's own personal values and the methodological norms--is readily apparent.

(b) Many writers agree that the therapist's values do, in fact, influence the patient. In one study it was discovered that according to 48 per cent of psychotherapists and psychoanalysts of the leading schools, "value concepts of the therapist do have and should have a direct influence upon the therapy"; according to 24 per cent an indirect influence was stated. (Wolff, (Buhler), 1962, pp. 11-12)

(c) In connection with the uncertainty in contemporary life regarding the validity of many transmitted values, one writer notes that "the 'collapse of values' and the general uncertainty in the field of value lead 'patients to apply' to their analysts 'for values which analysis cannot provide.'" (Wheelis, Buhler, 1962, p.13) This point is noteworthy since we may reasonably expect that the same uncertainties and shifts in contemporary values that are problematic for psychiatric patients may cause difficulties for analysts and therapists themselves in their own lives.

(d) It is noted that value-laden beliefs about persons form an integral part of different therapeutic approach, the author contends that "each person is a person of worth in himself and is therefore to be respected as such," and "each individual has the right of self-direction, to choose or select his own values and goals and to make his own decisions." (Patterson (Buhler), 1962, p.17) Buhler points out that this value placed on the individual worth of persons is naturally not limited to the nondirective school promoted by the author in question.

In concluding this section on methodological norms and value questions faced by therapists adhering to different therapeutic approaches, one final point deserves mention. The point can be made in the form of a metaquestion concerning the issues raised and discussed above: "Should the decision (on whether to take a stand on matters involving values) be left to the therapist's judgment, skill, and personal inclination? Or, should alternative solutions be studied and become part of our training?" (Buhler, 1962, p.21) It is apparent that there is a range of answers to this large question, each of them supported by various complex factors. Buhler's own position on this meta-issue does not take the form of a definite stand, but rather a recommendation for a program of research in the hope of obtaining a systematic and informed body of data on which to base a conclusion. (Buhler, 1962, pp. 26-27)

   (2) Values held by the analyst or therapist
       concerning his relationship with persons other
       than the patient himself (family, friends,
       employer, family physician, legal authorities,
       etc.)

In this category, the primary value questions faced by a therapist or analyst include moral decisions concerning whether or not to obtain or release information about his patient. It falls under the general area of doctor-patient confidentiality in medical ethics, but extends more widely into the legal and social arena in cases where the patient is presumed dangerous to others or judged likely to perform anti-social or destructive acts.

The issue of doctor-patient confidentiality is particularly acute in psychoanalytic and psychiatric contexts since the intimacy of the patient-psychiatrist relationship and the premium placed upon total honesty by the patient makes the therapist privy to a body of information about the patient shared perhaps by no one else. Thus when cases arise in which a therapist or analyst is asked about a patient, he may be faced

17

with a conflict between moral rules and conduct to which he generally subscribes (e.g., truthtelling), and the confidentiality imposed on him in his role as therapist by a professional code of ethics. A psychiatrist may be queried by a spouse who asks "What is going on with my wife (or husband)?" when the therapist knows that the patient has been having a series of extra-marital affairs. The parents of an unmarried daughter in college away from home may request information from a therapist about their daughter when the knowledge that she is living with her boyfriend would lead them to withdraw her financial support. A current or prospective employer might wish to have information about a patient in therapy, which, if known, would jeopardize present or future employment. In all such cases--and many others that might be cited--the professional code of ethics usually prevails and the psychiatrist withholds or even falsifies information to inquirers about the patient. The important point in this connection is that the therapist's decision must be viewed as a moral one. The answer is not simply "given" by citing the professional ethics governing the practice of psychoanalysis or psychotherapy. It is a genuine case of conflict of duty or obligation--one which might even be viewed as "built in" to the psychotherapeutic role. (Margolis, 1966, p.27)

There are other sorts of cases in which the conflict of duty facing a therapist has consequences that go beyond that of a personal moral dilemma. These are cases where a patient reveals information to his therapist about contemplated actions that will, if performed, have consequences injurious or fatal to other persons. Some years ago a case that received nationwide publicity concerned a person (under the care of a psychiatrist) who climbed up on a tower with a rifle and proceeded to pick off unsuspecting passers-by, killing several and maiming others. It was later revealed that the sniper had informed the psychiatrist of his intentions, or at least indicated his thought on the matter. In the face of a tendency to condemn the therapist for failure to inform the authorities about his patient's stated intentions, it should be remembered that it is not only the psychiatrist-patient privacy that is at stake, but also that the rights and freedom of the patient could be severely compromised if legal action were taken against him in the absence of any overt criminal act. This kind of case raises questions about professional competency to predict criminal acts or other deviant behavior performed by psychiatric patients--an issue which, although interesting and important, is peripheral to the concerns of this paper. (Livermore, etal, 1968, p. 80) It is apparent that the therapist's decision in this and similar cases is marked by fundamental moral concerns, involving not only the area of professional ethics but also those basic human rights that encompass privacy and freedom from interference--rights that may be violated if therapists revelaed certain information about their patients.

> (3) Value criteria implicit or explicit in psychiatric decisions concerning whom to treat.

This category of values concerns those directions that analysts and therapists are forced tomake about who should be helped by their services, given limited time and facilities for treating all persons who want to be treated or are in need of therapy. I want to exclude here those decisions based solely on professional judgment or evaluation of the need in a given case for treatment, since this area of values falls under III below. The area of concern in this section is a sub-problem of the broader issue in medical ethics concerning the allocation of time of medical personnel and equipment, where need or demand exceeds availability. It is a known fact that different socio-economic groups receive different medical care and treatment, both in the area of mental health and in medical practice as a whole. Often, where persons voluntarily seek psychiatric help, the therapist must make a decision about whom to treat--a decision based on the personal value system of the therapist and on his views about the social utility of helping some persons rather than others.

Closely connected with this issue--indeed, an integral part of it--are the financial considerations involved. The cost of private psychotherapy is exceedingly high and in the case of psychoanalysis, prohibitive for many persons who need or want treatment. Some analysts and therapists operate on a sliding financial scale related to the ability of patients to pay, but even this measure excludes large numbers of people. (Frank, 1961, p. 10)

19

The extent to which a therapist's own values enter
the picture in deciding whom to treat ranges from his
own preferences regarding what sort of problems he enjoys working with (e.g., psycho-sexual, underdeveloped
ego strength, sociopathic) to beliefs based on utili-
tarian considerations concerning which sorts of patients would be of most benefit to society or the
community if they were enabled to function better. The
former sorts of value judgments resemble appreciative
judgments regarding matters of taste whereas the latter
sort more closely approximate full-scale moral judgments of the sort "This person ought to be treated because...". where what follows the 'because' are reasons
that can be subsumed under some general moral rule. So
the values in this category are connected both with
matters of appreciation and taste on the part of the
therapist, and also with questions of social utility
and perceived benefit to community concerns reaching
beyond the mental health and well-being of the patient
himself. It is obvious that these values may conflict
with other sorts of ethical norms of justice or fiar-
ness, which enjoin that everyone has a right to psychotherapeutic help, no matter what the specific nature of
his disorder and no matter what social, intellectual,
or economic position he holds in society. The latter
moral constraint might entail the judgment that, ceteris
paribus, persons in need of treatment according to
generally accepted professional criteria should be
accepted on a first-come-first-served basis. On this
view, judgments of priority concerning whom to treat
when need exceeds availability of therapeutic time and
personnel would be based on degree of need of the patient, as assessed by competent psychotherapists.
(Frank, 1961, pp. 231-232)

There is no easy remedy for this state of affairs,
but apart from attempts at practical reform and systematic policy decisions, members of the psychotherapeutic
community would do well to examine their own criteria
for choosing or accepting patients and asking with
honesty and integrity whether the criteria they in fact
employ are consonant with their overall moral beliefs
concerning social justice.

III. Values implicit or explicit in various
psychiatric or psychotherapeutic theories

The overlap between values discussed in this section and those treated earlier is inevitable. The

20

focus in this section is on the way in which psychoanalytic and psychotherapeutic theories are themselves
value-laden. Since space does not permit an exhaustive
inquiry into all theories or even into all values explicit in some theories, the discussion will be confined to examples, falling under two broad sub-
categories.

A. Optimally functioning persons and "ideal types"

Most theories on which psychotherapeutic approaches
are based attempt to provide a background account that
purports to explain what goes wrong and when leading
to neurotic and psychotic disorders. In addition to
the theoretical terms, the empirical findings, and a
set of laws or law-like propositions, there is usually
an assumption--whether explicit or implicit--concerning
what type of functioning is desirable in a person.
This might be thought of, for the purpose of analysis,
as a sort of "ideal type" postulated by the theory.
Whether or not any actual persons embody this "ideal
type", comparative judgments can be made on the basis
of the degree to which the ideal type is approximated
in actual persons.

Perhaps one of the clearest and best-known examples of an ideal type is Freud's "genital ideal."
The notion is intimately bound up with Freud's developmental theory of infantile and childhood sexuality
in which the individual purportedly passes successively
through three early stages known as the oral, anal, and
phallic phases. Successfully passing through these developmental stages is a necessary condition for a-
chievement of "maturity", characterized in terms of the
"genital ideal", and adult neuroses and character disorders are attributable to unsuccessful passage from
one stage to the next, "arrest" or "fixation" at one
stage or another, "regression" to an earlier stage, and
other complications. The description of adult character types as "oral", "anal", or "phallic" derives from
this infancy-childhood explanatory scheme. The important point here is that these labels do not function
as mere descriptions, but contain a normative component.
The notion of the "genital ideal" serves as the ideal
of health and maturity in the adult person, and failure
to attain the ideal in accordance with the theoretical
suppositions is a mark of the individual's immaturity,
neurotic illness, character disorder, or the like.

21

Indeed, the locutions "anal character" and "oral personality" have crept into usage among informed (and even uninformed) lay persons, expressing negative value judgments when ascribed to individuals of their acquaintance.

It is not at all the purpose of the present inquiry to examine the correctness of the Freudian developmental theory its empirical testability, the breadth or narrowness of its application, etc. Although these and other issues are important and legitimate concerns, they are not central to the examination of the value questions under discussion here. The crucial point is that the notion of "genital ideal", as well as the "abnormal" character types, functions as a normative concept as well as a descriptive one in Freudian and neo-Freudian therapeutic judgments about persons' mental health and neuroses. Joseph Margolis points out that in developing his psychoanalytic theory, Freud used "a mixed model that shows clear affinities with the models that obtain in physical medicine and at the same time with the models of happiness and well-being that obtain in the ethical domain. (Margolis, 1966, pp. 81-82) This same issue arises in connection with values implicit in the models according to which mental disorders are classified, interpreted, and treated--in particular, with respect to the so-called "medical model". (Szasz, 1961) In the present context, our examination reveals that concepts comprising an integral part of the Freudian explanatory theory also play a normative role in characterizing the ideal of mental health or maturity, and enter into psychotherapeutic judgments of character disorder and neurotic illness. (Margolis, 1966, p.76)

Freud's psychoanalytic theory is sufficiently detailed and complex so that we might expect to find other examples of values embedded in the theory. Only one other instance will be cited here--an example that appears to embody the allegedly conflicting values of rationality and extreme hedonism (the "pleasure principle"). The example this time involves Freud's so-called "structural" concepts: id, ego, and superego. In view of Fritz Redlich, the following contradictory interpretations exist, each relating to different value considerations in Freud's theory.

One of the most quoted formulations

22

documenting Freud's belief in reason is the famous quotation 'Where the id was ego shall be.' The statement is taken by Fromm and also by many others as an expression of Freud's anti-instinctual viewpoint. It is interesting that Freud was also blamed for the opposite tendency, an immoral hedonism, and for the promotion of 'will' over intellect in the sense of Schopenhauer and Nietzsche. (Buhler, 1962, p.179)

It is not relevant for present purposes to try to resolve conflicting interpretations such as this, but rather to point out the extent to which value commitments infuse the theory in a manner of which Freud himself was undoubtedly unaware.

Turning now to another set of theories, we find some explicitly in the self-realization or self-actualization theories (to mention only a few, the theories of Erich Fromm, Karen Horney, Kurt Goldstein and Abraham Maslow). In all of these views, the value component is an essential part of the theoretical network. Fromm harks back to an Aristotelian conception of virtue in his self-realization theory of personality: "Fromm emphasizes that it is 'constant vigilance, activity, and effort' which 'can keep us from failing in the one task that matters: the full development of our powers within the limitations set by the laws of our existence.'" (Buhler, 1962, p.58)

Another representative of this group, Kurt Goldstin, couches his theory in terms of a " 'drive' that enables and impels the organism to actualize in further activities, according to its nature," holding that "optimal self-actualization also means health". (Buhler, 1962, p.58-59) And Abraham Maslow refers to a "Naturalistic 'value system' according to which the healthy person makes good choices. Desirability, health, and value are seen as closely related, if not identical." (Buhler, 1962, p.59) In all these theories, the role of the self-actualization principle is a dual one. It is descriptive of the process by which the self (a technical concept differing somewhat in each theory) develops and unfolds and fulfills its natural inclinations; it also functions in a normative role as the "ideal" or "optimum personality", toward which persons ought to strive and which characterizes the goal of successful psychotherapy.

This dual descriptive-normative role need not be viewed as a weakness of these (and other) theories, nor as an unwitting conflation of the two separate realms of facts and values. Indeed, what such examples serve to show is the way in which facts and values are often intertwined and how legitimate concepts and principles employed in theories may function doubly as descriptive or explanatory concepts, on one hand, and as normative concepts or principles on the other. (Macklin, 1968, pp. 400-409) If these self-actualization theories are to be faulted at all, it is not for their conflation of facts and values, but rather for their assumptions regarding man's "nature" and "inner self". The very principles which lead Fromm to adopt Aristotle's conception of man as having a unique and determinable nature. This conception has been subject to philosophical criticism for some time and it is unnecessary to repeat the arguments here. The point to be noted is only this: to the extent that self-realization theories rest on a conception of man's nature or "inner self", their underlying philosophical assumptions need to be examined. Charlotte Buhler appears to hold that this inquiry is largely an empirical matter. (Buhler, 1962, p.43)

She acknowledges that the concept of "natural inclinations" is problematic, but she apparently thinks it is a workable concept, satisfying the requirements of empirical significance. Thus, problems arise for self-realization theories at least to the extent that they presuppose uncritically some conception of man's nature or natural inclinations. But the problem must be seen to be not that of a conflation between facts and values, or descriptive and normative concepts, but rather one of empirical significance and testability of statements about fulfillment of self, achievement of potential, original tendencies, and the like.

Another set of theories that serve brief mention here is the group grounded in existential philosophy--in particular, Viktor Frankl's logotherapy approach. The predominant value in these theories is the development of man's "will to meaning" and its development in terms of a sense of responsibility. These theories have their basis primarily in the ethical precepts of philosophical existentialist theories. Buhler notes that according to existential psychiatric theories,

the existential self is not biologically determined.
(Buhler, 1962, p.59) These theories adhere to the
existentialist maxim that "existence precedes essence",
and hence they make no assumptions about man's nature
or natural inclinations. In accordance with existentialist theory, man "chooses" his self and is responsible for what he is and does. But where the self-
realization theories might be viewed as placing too
much emphasis on man's nature and potentiality, existential psychiatric theories appear to overemphasize
man's "ability to choose" and hence, to be responsible
for his character and conduct. The value in these
latter theories is placed, not on fulfillment or
actualization of one's potential, but on being "free
to choose" and achieving "meaning" in one's existence.

There are obviously a great number of psychiatric
and psychotherapeutic theories that have, of necessity,
been omitted from the above discussion. Nevertheless,
the account may serve to point out the different ways
in which different sorts of values are embedded implicitly in theoretical conceptions or made explicit
in the statement of a psychotherapeutic theory.

B.   Value suppositions concerning the aims and
     goals of psychotherapy

Closely connected with A, above, is a set of
value suppositions concerning the aims and goals of
psychotherapy itself. In some cases these values are
embedded in the psychotherapeutic theories themselves,
in other cases they emerge as consequences of the
application of a particular theory in psychotherapeutic
practice. An obvious point follows from the preceeding
discussion of ideal types and optimally functioning
persons. That is, to the extent that most theories embody a conception of mental health, optimally functioning personality or the like, the aims and goals of
therapy are set, the therapist strives to enable his
patient to achieve mental health, to function optimally, or to approximate the theory's ideal type. So
in the most obvious sense, the values inherent in the
aims and goals of psychotherapy lie in the success of
the therapy in achieving what the theory in question
holds to be optimal or desirable.

But there is another set of questions relating to
values in different psychotherapeutic systems. Among

these questions are the following: Should therapy be
concerned with eradicating mental illness and eliminating neuroses? Should it have a more positive goal,
e.g., to instill a set of beliefs and norms in persons
who are to be successfully treated? Should therapy
attempt to change behavior that, according to some
theory or other, is unfit, maladaptive, or aberrant?
Or should it aim at making persons happy, content,
fulfilled, whatever their behavior may be (that is,
even if their behavior is deviant or antisocial)?
These latter two questions presuppose two sets of
values which may at times conflict with one another:
(1) integration into the predominant group's value
system and behavior patterns (where the group in
question may be family, school, job, neighborhood,
subculture, or society in general); and (2) individual
happiness and well-being. Although these two sets of
values often go hand in hand, they sometimes diverge--
a fact perhaps increasingly evident in contemporary
American society with its divisions between youth and
their elders, radicals and Establishments, Black mili-
tants and the white community, etc. One writer who
reviewed the literature found a number of variables
according to which therapists evaluate the mental
health of their patients. He concluded from this
list that the variables in question delineate "the
desirable qualities of the rising young executive, of
the organization man,   or the upwardly mobile middle
class citizen." (Bloch, (Buhler), 1962, p.180) Need-
less to say, the values embodied in this conception
would be inimical to the value system and personal
goals of a radical youth, Black militant, a homosexual
artist, or any of a number of other persons who may
be in need of psychotherapy (for reasons other than
their failure or unwillingness to fit into the predominant social behavior patterns).

The value questions under consideration here
overlap to some extent with those discussed in section
II, namely, the therapist's own moral beliefs and value
preferences. But again, the emphasis here is on the
directives a therapist may receive from the psychotherapeutic system to which he subscribes. (Buhler,
1962, p.172) The distinction between objectives has
been put by one writer in terms of separation of the
"practical" and the "ideal" goals embodied by psychotherapeutic systems. (Wolberg, (Buhler, 1962,
p.173)) With some patients or according to some

theories, achievement of the practical goals is all
that is desired or required, whereas for other patients or according to other theories, therapy is not
considered successful unless the patient is able to
plan and act creatively and constructively.

SUMMARY AND CONCLUSION

This study has attempted to survey some of the
various ways in which questions and issues relating
to values enter into the theory and practice of psychotherapy and psychoanalysis. The analysis has been
provided by way of a classification schema distinguishing three chief categories of values, proceedings
from the more particular to the more general, with
the aim of obtaining a systematic and comprehensive
view of the issues and problems involved. There has
been little attempt here to suggest solutions to the
various difficulties encountered, since that task must
be left largely to theoreticians and practitioners in
the field. But the first step in any research program or practical reform is to see the issues involved in a clear and systematic manner, so philosophical analysis has its place, as always, in a field
where too little attention is given by practitioners
to analysis and criticism of their own commitments
and assumptions.

While I have not attempted to propound a unified
or overall thesis in this paper, I think that one
emerges from what has been examined and discussed.
That is, it seems more difficult than ever to maintain a fact-value distinction in a clear-cut or
systematic way. I do not claim that the distinction
can never be made, or that in some areas of inquiry
the lines are not clearly drawn. But in the area of
psychotherapy and psychoanalysis, values of various
sorts pervade the basic concepts, the theoretical
systems, the therapeutic methodology, and the psychopathological models that form the core of the theory
and practice. A number of examples were discussed
in which descriptive and normative conceptions are inextricably intertwined and cannot be separated without a degree of artificiality or ad hoc maneuvering.
In section III it was noted that a number of the central concepts in accounts such as psychoanalytic
theory and self-actualization theories possess an explicit or implicit normative force, as well as serving

as descriptive notions. Indeed, even in cases where a theoretical conception purports to be value-neutral or where a therapist tries to maintain "scientific neutrality", such efforts do not preclude the intrusion of value considerations.

There is no good reason to judge that the entrance of value considerations into psychotherapeutic theory and practice is pernicious or undesirable; what needs to be done is to clarify the multifarious ways in which this occurs. Theorists and clinicians alike need to examine with honesty their value assumptions and commitments with respect to their theoretical orientations, methodlological approaches, and therapeutic judgments. Only then can the meta-value judgment be made concerning which explicit or implicit values are worth maintaining and which ought to be eschewed. The price paid by a dogmatic adherence to scientific neutrality may be the erosion of those values most worth preserving.

BASIC CONCEPTS OF HUMANISTIC PSYCHOLOGY

Joseph E. Morris

Humanistic psychology is perhaps best described as a movement, a confluence of thought with philosophical origins in the existentialism of Heidegger, Kierkegaard, and Sartre and the phenomenology of Husserl. The strong subjective predisposition of these two philosophical approaches is conducive to the emergence of varied theoretical and operational expressions. This is a major reason for the eclectic character of humanistic psychology. It embraces an array of philosophical viewpoints including disciplines not confined to just psychology, counseling, or social work. On the surface, humanistic psychology appears to many as a diffuse and fragmented phenomenon. One prominent psychologist charged the movement "should not be seen as a license for vague or vapid thought" (Wertheimer, 1978, p. 744). In some quarters there may be justification for such observation. Nonetheless, the diversity and non-exclusiveness of humanistic psychology cannot be fairly characterized as theoretical anarchy, devoid of common themes. There are definite conceptual contours which shape the movement. The purpose of this article is to give them sharper definition and clarity.

Historical Overview

In 1954 Abraham Maslow compiled a mailing list with the following heading:

> For people who are interested in the scientific study of creativity, love, higher values, autonomy, growth, self-actualization, basic need, gratification, etc. (Sutich and Vich, 1969, p. 6)

This enchoate expression is perhaps the first general outline of humanistic psychology. Through the efforts of Anthony Sutich and Maslow, the Journal of Humanistic Psychology was first published in 1961 and in 1963 the American Association for Humanistic Psychology was formed. Both efforts placed emphasis upon an alternative to positivistic or behavioristic and classical psychoanalytic theories. They advocated theoretical approaches which would accentuate

creativity, self-growth, self-actualization, identity
formation, individual autonomy, value orientation,
responsibility, and other personality variables heretofore deemphasized or omitted from other psychological initiatives. In 1965 Frank T. Servin published
Humanistic Viewpoints in Psychology. From a broad
spectrum of contributors Severin organized the articles to reflect three areas of major emphasis: (1)
unity of personality, self-determination and the primacy of self; (2) a serious re-evaluation of methodology in producing techniques applicable to immediate
experience and a review of the assumptions underlying
the methodology; and (3) discussions related to values,
inner dynamics of creativity, and self-actualization.
Other advocates joining this attempt to delineate
the basic principles of the new movement were James
F.F. Bugental (1965, 1967) and Anthony Sutich and
Miles Vich (1969).

Two significant events occurred in 1970. A new
subdivision called the Division of Humanistic Psychology was created within the American Psychological
Association. In August of that year the First International Congress of Humanistic Psychology convened
at the New University of Amsterdam. Following this
assembly a consensus of basic theoretical concepts
slowly emerged. As President of the Congress,
Charlotte Bühler fused these concepts into unified expression and further elaborates upon them in conjunction with Melaine Allen (1972). The following
condensed list of those concepts (Cf. Morris, 1979,
1980) characterizes the approaches of such mainstream
psychologists as Carl Rogers, Rollow May, Abraham
Maslow, Charlotte Bühler, and Adrian Van Kaam, to
mention a few:

1. Emphasis upon the whole person as a model,
importance of the individual self, and the uniqueness
of persons.
2. A positive theoretical model of persons as
active, free, and responsible.
3. A theory of knowledge based upon immediate
experience.
4. The self as a central core system of personality; intentionality as basic to self-discovery.
5. Values oriented to life goals; self-
actualization; and self-transcendence.

6. Creativity as a universal human characteristic.

Analysis of Basic Concepts

Wholeness, individuality, and uniqueness of persons. Humanistic psychology maintains that "the central core of personality consists in its unity and uniqueness" (Severin, 1965, p. 3). Maslow and Rogers followed the lead of Kurt Goldstein's (1940) application of Gestalt perceptual theory to personality and motivation. A basic presupposition of Goldstein's theory was the aspiration of human personality toward unity and wholeness, in contrast to trait theories of behavioral psychologists who tended to compartmentalize personality. Traits are not isolated bits of personality which can be studied piecemeal. They are parts of an interrelated, patterned whole organized by a central core "self" which reflects the uniqueness of personality. For humanists the whole is greater than the sum of its parts. Individuals actualize their potential to become more than they actually are. An essential aspect of this concept for some humanists, especially Maslow, is emphasis upon positive, wholesome attributes such as attitudes of love, happiness, trust, etc., rather than preoccupation with the failings and weaknesses of human nature.

This holistic approach includes the recent emphasis in humanistic psychology upon the essential unity of mind and body. The two are inseparable. Cartesian dualism, Rene Descartes' fundamental division of reality into two separate realms, is rejected. Holistic application to health is paralleled in physics by the replacement of Newtonian reductionism with the quantum understanding of a dynamic universe. Human personality is no longer viewed as a machine composed of many parts, but rather as an organic, dynamic whole. Recent research in the fields of psychophysiology, neurophysiology, neurochemistry, and psychoneurology provide empirical data supporting the theoretical presuppositions of this holistic orientation. An entire new field of holistic medicine has emerged encompassing practitioners who, through the use of biofeedback, brainwave training, mental imagery, transcendental meditation, hypnosis, etc., are demonstrating the delicate, intricate interrelations of mind and body.

31

Positive, free and responsible humanity. A positive view of humans as active mediators of their own existence is universal with humanistic psychologists. This notion stems logically from their philosophical presupposition that the natural state of human existence is one of freedom. Freedom is a precondition to the creation of one's self-becoming. Persons are free to become what they choose. In Jean-Paul Sartre's words we become our choices, and Rollo May (1961a) adds, "within the limits of our given world" (p. 13). Individuals are agents of decision and, therefore, responsible for their decisions.

Humanists do not deny the combined influences of genetic predisposition, constitution, historical circumstance, and environmental factors upon the development of personality. They accept the reality of these forces. They do insist, however, upon a

> thin margin of freedom we have when we
> react to, and attempt to exploit, the
> given, usually unalterable, conditions
> of our lives....(Shaffer, 1978, p. 15)

This "thin margin of freedom" is what May alludes to as "the limits of our given world," what Heidegger referred to as our existential "Throwness." Victor Frankl (1959) speaks of this notion of freedom in From Death Camp to Existentialism, the result of his years in a concentration camp. For him life was shaved down to the bare edge of existence. All else became meaningless, except the freedom to choose one's attitude toward one's fate. Rogers infers the same inner freedom, something which exists in the person aside from outward choices or options.

Related to this model of persons as active, free, and responsible is the notion that individuals are in a constant process of becoming. May (1961b) points out that the word existence comes from the Latin root existere, which means literally "to stand out, emerge" (p. 12). All of the major representatives of humanistic psychology acknowledge this fundamental thesis in their writings. Perhaps nowhere does it receive greater expression and emphasis than in Rogers' (1961) On Becoming a Person:

> Life at its best, is a flowing, changing

> process in which nothing is fixed...guided
> by a changing understanding of and interpre-
> tation of my experience. It is always in
> process of becoming. (p. 27)

As the individual becomes immersed in the process, the
inner reference to meanings becomes more accurate.
The results are greater feelings of freedom and
acceptance of the "fluid process of experiencing,
using it comfortably as a major reference for behavior" (p. 157). One of the end results of this experience is an increased sense of self-responsibility.

Knowing is experiencing. Related and integral to
the preceding concepts is the assumption by humanists
that the experience of human existence is imperative
for humanistic concept formation. Experience is the
only trustworthy basis for the individual's knowledge
of self. And the only way the individual can know
reality is to be involved experientially in it, i.e.,
as a participant in relationship with it:

> There is no such thing as truth of reality
> for a living human being except as he par-
> ticipates in it, is conscious of it and
> has some relationship to it. (May, 1961a,
> p. 14)

With this Kierkegaardian statement May expresses
the phenomenological concept that reality lies in the
individual's experience of the event and not in the
isolated objective event. Phenomenology is the
description of the data, the "givens" of immediate
experience. It involves the effort to experience
the phenomena as expressed in reality. The approach
is not to explain but rather to understand phenomena.

A digression at this point is in order on the
relationship of phenomenology to existentialism.
Some questions have arisen regarding the marriage of
existential principles to phenomenology, reviving the
conflict between freedom and determinism. The controversy centers on the terms "phenomenal field" and
"phenomenal self."

The phenomenological model most noted in psychology today is that expounded by Syngg and Combs.
Ultimately, they declare that the phenomenal field

33

holds primacy over the self, a form of determinism
implying no choice for the individual:

> ...we might say that the individual is en-
> gaged in a continuous process of making
> "choices." As a matter of fact, no choice
> whatever exists. He attempts that which
> appears to him self-enhancing and attempts
> to avoid that which appears to him as
> threatening. What he does is dependent upon
> the differentiations he can make in his
> phenomenal field. (Snygg and Combs, 1949,
> quoted in Beck, 1963, p. 66)

Humanists propose the opposite. The phenomenal self
"chooses" what and where to perceive in the phenomenal
field, presupposing freedom of the organism. This
will be discussed more fully in the following section
on intentionality.

May (1961a), Rogers (1951), and Maslow (1966)
see no incongruence in their application of phenomenological epistemology to existential principles. Employment of phenomenology does not necessarily imply
a deterministic theoretical framework. They seem
more concerned with methodology rather than a
"shotgun" marriage to philosophical ideology. For
this reason they avoid embroilment over some of the
finer nuances of philosophy and its relationship to
actual therapeutic application.

The self and intentionality. As indicated
earlier, humanistic psychologists unite in their
shared view that the self is a "core system" which
serves as the focal point of the individual's goal
setting. They contend that the psychoanalytic
position presents the self as an object and refrains
from considering it as a primary psychological unit.
May (1961a) counters this notion:

> Autonomy by its very nature can be located
> only in the centered self....My self, or my
> being (the two at this point are parallel)
> is to be found at the center at which I
> know myself as the one responding....The
> point I wish to make is that being must be
> presupposed in discussions of ego and iden-
> tity and that the centered self must be
> basic to such discussions. (pp. 34-35)

Rogers (1959) refers to the self as "a fluid and changing gestalt, a process, but at any given moment it is a specific entity" (p. 200). In a semantical preference, Bugental (1965) chooses the concept "I": "...irreducibly a unity...the essential being. Only the "I" is truly the subject in the world....All other entities are objects" (pp. 201-202).

This consciousness of being, the self, expresses itself and receives its identity through the dynamics of intentionality. For phenomenologists (especially Husserl and Bretano, his teacher) intentionality is an innate quality of consciousness. The two are inherently bound. As May expresses it (1969), "consciousness is defined by the fact that it intends something, points toward something outside itself--specifically, that it intends the object" (p. 226), "phenomenal self" supercedes "phenomenal field."

Intention is an act of outreach and purpose. One's purposes in life, those which give life meaning, are achieved through intentionality. Freedom, choice, decision, and responsibility are all deeply interwoven into intentionality. The way one chooses to relate to the world is a reflection of one's intentions. Existentially speaking, the action is the intention and the intention is the action, the two being inseparable. We may or may not be aware of the intentions underlying our actions. Nevertheless, within the humanistic/existential conceptual framework we bear responsibility for our "choices" and "decisions." The end result is authentic existence. As Bugental noted (1965), "man's intentionality is the basis of his identity" (p. 12). Persons become truly human and experience their identity in the crucible of decision (Cf. Tillich, 1952). In a reversal of Socrates' ancient dictum, "to know the good is to do the good," humanists might state, "to do the good is to know the good." The following statement by Charlotte Bühler (1967) summarizes the humanist position on the interrelationship between self and intentionality:

> In other words, I believe that certain basic tendencies interact and are integrated in this core system. I called these basic tendencies need-satisfaction, self-limiting adaptation, creative expansion, and upholding the internal order. This core system's

thrust into life is that intentionality
with which the individual strives toward a
hoped for fulfillment. In the ideal case,
this is identical with the realization of
the individual's best potentials. (p. 43)

This basis assumption leads directly into the next
fundamental concept of humanistic psychology: healthy
humans want to create values.

Values, goals, and self-actualization. Humanistic psychologists reject the principle of homo-
stasis which depicts individuals as maintaining or
restoring an inner balance to reduce tensions. Instead they opt for an open-ended system of personality. They contend that the core system of self
and intentionality moves with purpose toward the fulfillment of potential, as suggested by Buhler avove.
Their focus is upon goals, self-realization, and self-
actualization. Karen Horney (1950) and Erich Fromm
(1941) first promoted the term self-realization. Self-
actualization was proposed by Kurt Goldstein (1939)
and fully developed by Maslow (1954). In a similar
vein Victor Frankl (1965) introduced the term self-
transcendence, "a constitutive characteristic of being
human that always points and is directed to something
other than itself" (p. 113).

Though some leading humanists quibble about
nuances implied by these terms, their differences of
interpretation seem more semantical than qualitative.
In essence, all are promoting the same concepts of
goal orientation, goal fulfillment, and self-growth.
Individuals, through a growing awareness of themselves
and the world around them, begin to activate their
potentials with the purpose of bringing them to actualization or realization. In so doing they achieve fulfillment in life. Buhler (1967), Frankl (1955), and
Maslow (1962) all feel that self-realization in self-
transcendent goals is experienced as "meaningful"
life. Healthy individuals express themselves creatively in the pursuit of these goals.

Creativity. The concept of creativity as a universal human characteristic is presupposed by all of
the major proponents of humanistic psychology and relates in some way to each of the concepts discussed
above. Buhler (1972) gives creativity a primary role,

36

calling it "the most central concept of humanistic psychology" (p. 59). Reflecting on his own research, Maslow (1954) was one of the first to emphasize that the most "universal characteristic of all the people studied or observed was their creativeness" (p. 223). Creativity is viewed as fundamental to human nature, an innate potentiality shared by all persons.

The humanist understanding of creativity reflects their interpretation of reality as process and human personality as an open system with "certain freedoms of operation and potentials for change" (Bühler, 1971, p. 51). The relationship of this ontology to the tricky problem of predictability in science is significant. May (1961a) addresses the issue.

> Although the healthy person is "predictable" in the sense that his behavior is integrated and he can be depended upon to act according to his own character, he always at the same time shows a new element in his behavior. His actions are fresh, spontaneous, interesting; and in this sense he is just the opposite of the neurotic and his predictability. This is the essence of creativity. (p. 31).

The humanist feels that the "real" person is not subject to rigid prediction. Therefore, the goals of psychotherapy are neither precise predictability nor control. Successful psychotherapy is inversely proportionate to reduction of control and predictability because of the increase in spontaneity and creativity. Humans are the active mediators, the creators, of their existence.

Subjectivity

The preceding six major concepts of humanistic psychology emerge from a deeper and more fundamental philosophical hermeneutic: subjectivity. The revolt against the traditional scientific methodologies, based upon empiricism and a passion for objective verifiability, has given the role of subjectivity fresh posture.

The meaning of subjectivity for humanists has double significance. First, it is a justification

for their approach toward a new definition of science:
"It is indeed in the matrix of immediate personal subjective experience that all science, and each individual scientific research, has its origins" (Rogers,
1965, p. 165). Van Kaam (1965) concurs with Rogers:
"Important in the development of science is the
realization that science is relatively subjective"
(p. 175). Secondly, subjectivity defines the natural
state of the self vis-a-vis the real world:

> There is a quality of living subjectively in
> the experience, not feeling about it....The
> self, at this moment, is this feeling. This
> is being in the moment, with little self-
> conscious awareness....The self is, subjec-
> tively, in the existential moment. (Rogers,
> 1961, p. 147)

Humanistic epistemology, alluded to earlier, begins
with conscious experience. This pehnomenological approach establishes conscious experience as the basis
of knowledge about the world and others. The behaviorists' regard for "causes" is rejected. Subjective consciousness interprets reality in its own
right and is accepted as valid for each individual.
This provides the framework for empathic understanding
of various viewpoints and perceptions; that reality is
not so much an objective given, as it is subjectively
perceived by different individuals.

CONCLUSION

The close interrelation of all of the humanistic
concepts is evident. They are part of a dynamic philosophical network, where thought in one area necessarily triggers thought in all. The order of their presentation is really insignificant. Creativity, self-
actualization, intentionality, self, experiential
knowledge, responsibility, becoming, individuality,
wholeness--all are contingent upon and logically relate to each other. Humanistic psychology, within the
subjective framework, maintains a coherent belief
system, with little resemblance to "vague or vapid
thought." Correctives and deterrents to the development of dogma or ideology are self-contained within
the meaning of the basic concepts. Rigid elitist
elements--the humanistic movement contains its fair
share--are common to any evolution of thought. But as
Shaffer (1978) points out, "humanistic orientation in

38

psychology...will hopefully exist for as long as there are theorists who believe in the importance of the individual and human consciousness.

Hopefully, a review of the basic concepts of humanistic psychology will increase understanding and acceptance of its diversity and flexibility. Its commitment to principles of empathy and openness is a reflection of integrity, a congruence of philosophy and practice. Admittedly, this approach significantly reduces control and predictability, attracting umbrage and skepticism from some scientific quarters. But the dividends in creativity and expansion of potentiality are equally significant.

In a closing comment Charlotte Bühler (1979), shortly before her death, addressed this "awakening to new potentialities" and the future role of humanistic psychology:

> As I see it now, what happened (and still happens) is that we have been and still are contributing to a wide-spread process that is going on in the Western World. It might be called an awakening to new potentialities, individually as well as socially. It is the awakening of a new type of consciousness of inner forces as well as of human possibilities for social living. Humanistic psychology partly helps: it partially reflects this process. (p. 5)

NON-SCIENTIFIC SOURCES
OF PSYCHOTHERAPEUTIC APPROACHES

Robert N. Sollod

Psychotherapeutic approaches purport to be scientific both in their underlying conceptions and in the methods of their development and validation. This view has a legitimizing function as it places the psychotherapies within the prestigious aura of psychology and the natural sciences. The model of psychotherapy as an application of science has served to facilitate its institutionalization within the academic world. The notion that the psychotherapies are scientific is also a way of encouraging some useful activities such as the accumulation of knowledge through the exchange of information by communities of investigators and the exploration of the unknown leading to the possible improvement of human life. Many considerations, however, lead to the conclusion that the psychotherapies do not constitute an applied science within the discipline of psychology. Among such considerations are the fragmentation of the psychotherapies into a variety of contending approaches with vastly different conceptions and methodologies and the rapid rise-and-fall of therapeutic trends. The subjective and value-laden aspects of the development and validation of the psychotherapies is in marked contrast to the formulations of positivistic science (Ayer, 1959; Nagel, 1961; Popper, 1958).

One crucial but questionable aspect of the view that psychotherapy is an applied science is the appeal to empirical validation or verification. This argument states that to the extent that psychotherapeutic approaches submit to empirical investigation and demonstrate effectiveness, their underlying theories can be considered scientifically demonstrated to be valid. Such a conclusion has had an important place in the history of psychotherapy's institutionalization, for it was through empirical outcome research that Rogers was able to bring client-centered therapy within university psychology programs. Subsequently, other approaches have attained apparent scientific status through the process of empirical validation.

Rogers' case for the institutionalization of

psychotherapy within psychology as an applied science was based on two considerations: the first, derived from Goodwin Watson's findings, was that his approach was in some way universal as it represented a distillation of the common elements of psychotherapy practiced by many therapeutic schools (Watson, 1940), and the second was that the effectiveness of client-centered therapy could be empirically validated. Thus psychotherapy would be analogous to the applied science of agriculture, with which Rogers was very familiar, in that the results of various techniques could be empirically tested. (Sollod, 1978).

In regard to the claim to scientific status based on the presumed universality of non-directive approaches, it can be pointed out that the mere prevalence or acceptance of an approach in no way justifies or indicates its scientific validity. Furthermore, psychotherapy has long drawn from directive approaches with quite contrary assumptions about personality. Hypnosis, suggestion, and confrontation, ignored by Watson and Rogers, have also subsequently been demonstrated to be effective techniques. Thus, the non-directive approach, though based on fashionable therapeutic modalities, represented only one stream of psychotherapeutic practice and could not properly claim universality.

The second contention, which is at the heart of psychotherapy's institutionalization within the discipline of psychology, merits careful examination.

<u>Critique</u> <u>of</u> <u>the</u> <u>empirical</u> <u>validation</u> <u>argument</u>.

Using empirical validation of therapeutic effects as an indication of the scientific status of psychotherapy or as a scientific demonstration of the validity of the theory and associated methods is fallacious. Such a reliance on empirical verification to determine the truth of a given theory has been questioned in recent formulations of scientific methodology (Toulmin, 1969). By no means can the investigation of a procedure within a framework of empirical methodology demonstrate that the truth of the underlying theory is scientifically demonstrated. In fact, a procedure based on a <u>non-scientific</u> theory may be investigated and perhaps demonstrated to be effective in causing change.

The pragmatic value of a given method may be demonstrated, but an empirical demonstration of its clinical effectiveness in no way demonstrates the truth of the theory underlying the technique. In the case of client-centered therapy, an entire comprehensive theory of personality is considered validated by empirical research, yet only certain facets of the method (or merely social influence) may actually account for the observed effects. In Freudian theory certain techniques such as free association may potentiate the therapeutic process, yet the whole theory's truth is considered substantiated by outcome research or clinical observation. Studies of the effectiveness of systematic desensitization, a behavioral method, have demonstrated that such a technique is effective in the treatment of certain conditions such as phobias, but the efficacy of the techniques in no way validates a behavioral description of personality or even demonstrates that there is an actual process of desensitization (Wachtel, 1977).

In addition, a self-fulfilling aspect may be operative in outcome tests of psychotherapeutic theories. Such an effect further vitiates the validity of using empirical evaluation of effects as an indication of the truth of the underlying approach. Wachtel (1977) has noted that, unlike the physical world, other people are not non-reactive. "How they behave toward us is very much influenced by how we behave toward them, and hence by how we initially perceive them. Thus, our initial (in a sense distorted) picture of another person can end up being a fairly accurate predictor of how he or she will act toward us because, based on our expectation that the person will be hostile, or accepting, or sexual, we are likely to act in such a way as to eventually draw such behavior from the person and thus have our (initially inaccurate perception 'confirmed.'" pp. 54-55).

Extrapolating this concept into the psychotherapeutic situation, it becomes apparent that the therapist, who occupies an influential position in the life of the patient, can exert a marked impact on the patient's behavior in line with the predictions of the therapist's theory. Such an impact could be mediated, for example, through suggestion, choice of

interpretation, and differential support or lack of
support for certain of the patient's behaviors.
Analysts, who usually have a skeptical attitude toward rapid change, particularly in early stages in
therapy, will be more likely to take a different stance
toward such change than will behaviorists or client-
centered therapists, who fully expect the patient to
have the power to change significantly in a brief
time. No doubt, such therapeutic stances affect the
actual behavior of the patient.

Therapists, moreover, rarely use the experience
of patients who do not improve to disconfirm their
psychotherapeutic theories. They usually find other,
more acceptable explanations, including the severity
or nature of the patient's pathology or, perhaps, the
patient's lack of motivation. In the concept of
"negative therapeutic reaction", the lack of positive
response may be seen as a confirmation of the underlying psychotherapeutic theory. Another possible
explanation is that the therapeutic theory and method
were correct but that the therapist failed in its
application (Sandler et. al., 1970).

A further consideration is that the therapist
should believe in a given theory and convey such a
belief in order to enhance the effectiveness of
therapy. The therapist's belief in a therapeutic
approach is considered a major aspect of the Placebo,
or non-specific therapeutic effect (Frank, 1973;
Shapiro, 1971). In addition, some therapeutic theory
is required by the therapist to provide a sense of
order regarding the complexities of the patient's
behavior and experiences and to guide his or her own
responses. The therapist is not, as a consequence, in
a favorable position to question those very theories
on which he or she must rely to function effectively.

The use of the effectiveness of therapeutic
approaches as an indication of the truth of an
underlying therapeutic paradigm thus appears to be
more similar to the types of testing which a variety
of non-scientific paradigms are subject to than it is
to the process of scientific verification. For example, a person may validate a religious belief or
theory because of its innate appeal, its compatibility
with the experiences and observations of the individual, its power to reorder the believer's experience,
and as a result of its perceived beneficent impact

44

on the adherent's life and that of others. Likewise, an artist may have a useful motivating conception of reality which underlies his or her work, or an educator may draw on certain educational philosophies or views of human nature. These non-scientific areas are analogous to psychotherapy in their dual emphasis upon the necessity for a comprehensive view of reality--essentially untestable by scientific means--and the requirement of a certain utility or practical effect. As do psychotherapeutic approaches, they may also claim unique insight, truth, usefulness, or comprehensiveness, but they have little pretension to scientific validity. The comprehensiveness, coherence, or effectiveness of a theory in no way ensures its scientific status.

Development and institutionalization of psychotherapeutic forms.

Instead of the ongoing development, testing and reformulation of a few theories typical of science, psychotherapy presents a proliferation of forms and methods. Transactional analysis, gestalt therapy, primal scream therapy, psychosexual therapy, encounter groups, reality therapy, and assertive training as well as many other approaches all have a cadre of enthusiastic practitioners and adherents. There is no unifying theory underlying these approaches, and the attempts to study empirical outcomes often lead to the validation of discrepant or contradictory theories. The psychotherapies do not resemble a science either in terms of their development of theories and methods or in their organization as a discipline.

In general, psychotherapeutic forms have opted, as have behavior therapy and client-centered therapy, to be institutionalized within the discipline of psychology or, as has psychoanalysis, to develop their own institutional structures. Behavior therapy is the purest example of the former pattern. It fits the definition of a scientific endeavor more adequately than other therapeutic forms as it rests to a large extent on laboratory experiments and relies on the accumulated observations and experiments of numerous investigators according to specified methodologies (Krasner, 1971). Behavior therapy is not, however, as pure an applied science as it purports to be. Its choice of goals and methods is greatly affected by cultural considerations, and its techniques are often not as closely grounded in empirical research as they superficially appear to be. Systematic desensitization, a predominant technique, is, for example, presumably based on animal research findings but has the added ingredient of subjective imagery. This innovation appears to have been added de novo for its clinical impact and was not derived directly from behavioral theory. The recent cognitive revolution in behavioral therapy was justified more by clinical pragmatism than by either behavioral theory or by an accumulation of empirical research (Wolpe, 1980). Furthermore, as in other therapeutic forms, the collection and development of effective techniques by no means ensures either that the techniques work for the theoretically supposed reasons or that the theories underlying the techniques have been demonstrated to be true.

A second course adopted by the psychoanalytic schools and a wide variety of other approaches, has been to develop their own institutional structures outside of either university or medical school environments. Such structures facilitate the transmission and development of elaborate clinical procedures and theories, but they insulate the disciplines from modification due to advances in the basic sciences or to systematic empirical evaluation. The lack of emphasis on outcome research and the reliance on case history material as well as the plethora of different theories, all eagerly espoused by their adherents, indicates that these institutionalized forms do not represent scientific traditions but rather clinical disciplines which have drawn on certain aspects of biological science or psychology in the formulation of their approaches. Unlike scientific endeavors, they have not devoted much effort to testing their assumptions or modifying them as a result of empirical findings. It has recently been proposed that the psychoanalytic world has not developed any agreed upon systematic procedures for evaluating difficult issues in the field (Wolitzky and Silverman, 1980). The existence of such procedures to resolve disputes is vital to any endeavor which purports scientifically to base its conclusions on the cumulative theorizing and investigating activity of many participants.

The weakness of the empirical validation

argument for the scientific status of the psychotherapies as well as a brief consideration of the
course of their development and the pattern of their
institutionalization lead to the conclusion that although the psychotherapies purport to be scientific,
their actual nature is veiled by such a label. By
habitually thinking of the therapies as scientific,
we are inclined to ignore the influence of non-
scientific factors such as culture, history, and
personality on their origins and development. If the
psychotherapies are not forms of applied science, we
are left with the question of how best to define them
and how most adequately to comprehend their sources
and functions.

The link between religion and psychotherapy.

The concept of gnosis, which has been a stream
of thought and practice within many religions, is
that the individual can reach a state of purity and
enlightenment through an arduous process of abstinence and acquisition of self-knowledge, usually
under the guidance of those who had previously been
initiated into the mysteries of esoteric knowledge
(Hixon, 1978). The Delphic injunction, "Know thyself
everywhere and always," has been the keystone of a
proliferation of gnostic approaches throughout history. It can be found in sources ranging from the
Mahayanan Buddhist emphasis on self-observation and
Gurdjieff's emphasis on self-remembering (Riordan,
1975) to the work of the ancient Alchemists (Burkhardt,
1967). As the amount of wisdom available to human-
kind is considered limited in the light of gnostic
thought, only a highly qualified few are chosen to
undertake this process. Nor is gnostic effort intended to lead directly to beneficent change in outer
life but rather to reveal to the aspirant an inner
certitude unavailable to the rest of humanity. The
discipleship relationship is usually seen as necessary within such forms, and the reactions of the disciple to the Master are used to promote self-
knowledge.

Freudian psychoanalysis (as well as Jungian)
has within it many features which resemble gnostic
practice as well as a residue of elements of Judaic
religiosity. Patienthood is restricted to that elite
most qualified in terms of intellect, character and

economic means for the task of exhaustive self-examination. One can comment on the rigorous process required of those who are to become analysts as well as the necessity that this process be carried out under the guidance of a person previously "initiated." Therapeutic neutrality and abstinence, as in gnosticism, are also important parts of the analytic process. Freud (1919) stated that, "analytic treatment should be carried through, as far as is possible, under privation--in a state of abstinence." Theoretically psychoanalysis is predicated, as is gnosticism, on the notions that human beings are the servants of forces outside of their ordinary consciousness and that knowledge is hidden from the untrained mind. Judaic aspects of psychoanalysis are also discernible (Bakan, 1958). The interpretation of the meaning of the patient's statements with attention paid to the slightest nuances as a clue to hidden significance is emphasized in a manner most similar to Talmudic interpretation. Truth, is not seen as suddenly revealed but worked for through a careful searching process.

Rogerian therapy stands in contrast to the Freudian approach. Its emphasis is on the individual's growing understanding of his or her feelings. The therapist, in this approach, is a facilitator of the patient's discovery of his or her true self (Rogers, 1961). The therapist's effectiveness does not occur primarily as a result of a refined intellect or of having completed an arduous initiatory process but rather as a function of an attitude of unselfish, disinterested caring and love (termed "accurate empathy and unconditional positive regard"), which in a Christian framework could be considered as forms of agape. The Rogerian emphases share with gnosticism a seeking after the true self and a desire to have a more superficial sense of reality behind. Rogers is also similar in emphasis to Protestant Christianity with its stress on individual responsibility and individual emotional commitment as well as its belief in the healing power of love. As Vitz (1977) has pointed out, however, the goal of Rogers' approach is not God or Christ but rather an actualization of the individual's own quite secular self. The client-centered emphasis on each person working out his or her own destiny without the interference of others, the trust in feeling and in intuition to guide this process, and the emphasis on present-time orientation is in line with the teachings of many Protestant writers.

Rogers' background is relevant to understanding the deeply Protestant style of his therapeutic approach. The details of his background have been described elsewhere in greater detail (Sollod, 1978), but the main features can be presented here. According to autobiographical writings (Rogers, 1961), he came from a strictly ascetic and religious family in which there was no drinking, dancing, card-playing, theater-going, and little social life. He decided to become a minister in college and went on a World student Christian Federation Conference to China at the age of 20. During this time he broke away from the traditional religious views of his parents. He completed the first year of Union Theological Seminary, a liberal institution, but was unhappy with the dogmatism he perceived even in such a liberal environment and switched to the goal of becoming a clinical psychologist at Teachers' College, Columbia University. His rejection of the ministry did not consist of a rejection of Christian values, but rather of the dogmatism he believed to be associated with the ministerial role. There is evidence that, even prior to his entering graduate school in psychology, he had anticipated many aspects of non-directive therapy in his participation in developing a leaderless group at Union Theological Seminary.

The typically non-authoritarian relationship between therapist and client is analogous to the relatively informal clergy-laity distinction among Protestants. The client-centered therapist is saying, in effect, to the patient, "I want to help you to work out your destiny as you see fit, according to your own light. You will find your path as you learn to trust your feelins and experiences." The Protestant style of client-centered therapy stands out even more sharply by contrast with the almost rabbinic-gnostic quality of psychoanalysis. Here the thrust is in the trained reason of the therapist and his or her mastery of the almost Talmudic interpretive art. The patient is expected to apprehend his or her behavior in the light of reason, balanced by the experience incorporated in tradition as expressed through institutionally approved authority.

49

The temporal emphasis is on the past or on interpreting the present in light of the past. The analyst, in effect, says to the patient, "We will apply
reason to your life so that you may understand your-
self and you will know what to do."

The parallels between psychotherapeutic and
religious forms strongly suggest that many psychotherapeutic approaches are largely derivations of
traditional forms. These cultural derivatives occur
in post-traditional industrializing society yet nonetheless contain within them many of the elements of
religion. Differing perspectives on this phenomenon
can be offered. From the point of view of societal
history and development, the newer psychotherapeutic
forms can be seen as having the function of serving
the psychological (and sociological) needs previously
served by religions. From the religious point of
view, the development of psychotherapy must be seen
as extremely detrimental to the extent that psychotherapeutic forms may respond to and satiate religious
motivations such as the wish for enlightenment or salvation. From a religious point of view, such motivation must be considered part of humanity's spiritual
potential and not merely a psychological need. To aid
in clarifying this problem, it is important for psychologists to begin to sort out what aspects of their
approaches represent a form of substitute religion,
closely mimicking religious traditions and often drawing on those very motivations which may lead to religious commitment and spiritual development. Quite
possibly, the very appeal of therapeutic forms is
based on their similarity to those religious and
cultural elements with which people are familiar,
although with a more secular content. A fundamental
analysis of the religious and scientific bases of
various psychotherapeutic approaches would lead to the
clarification of many of the ethical issues on the
interface between psychotherapy and religion. Berger
(1977) has commented on the sociological and socio-
historical functions of psychotherapy, particularly
psychoanalysis. He has theorized that the psychotherapeutic movement and modern psychologism support
the role and identity of the individual in an industrialized, modern society while at the same time
facilitating the social control of the individual. In
the current presentation, the psychotherapies are
seen as having religious forms but secular contents;

they are thus viewed as serving the role of midwife for the process of cultural evolution from traditional religious societies to an industrialized, secular one. In their role as cultural midwife, the therapies facilitate the development of the individual self as the basis from which action springs and support the individual's contacting his or her feelings as one basis for action, whereas the traditional religions emphasized a deference and respect for those authorities and religious beliefs upon which an individual might depend and on the repression of individual feelings.

Rogerian therapy can be viewed as a therapeutic form enabling people brought up with a firm grounding in religion, family, and community to adjust to the new freedoms and opportunities of the Post WW II era. The solution provided in client-centered therapy was to focus on feelings in the here and now, to aim for constant growth and change in response to the changing circumstances of life. Such an approach would not be useful for those who are unsure of their basic values or who are locked-into fixed roles and patterns of adjustment. (Sollod, 1978).

Certain aspects of Freudian approaches, likewise, may be seen as a means of facilitating adjustment from the Victorian world and a traditional ghetto society to a more secular existence. Certainly, Freud redefined sexuality in such a way that the Victorian assumptions about human nature were challenged.[1] The use of the concept of transference in clinical practice frees the individual to function in a secular world without being encumbered by child-like attitudes and feelings toward others. In a traditional ghetto (as well as Victorian) society, it was quite appropriate to view elders as father figures and experience

---

[1]An interesting observation is the psychoanalysis is becoming increasingly popular in the developing countries of South America, which are currently experiencing a transition from traditional notions of sexual morality to a more modern view of sexuality. This trend is occurring at the same time that psychoanalysis is on the wane in Western Europe and North America, where such a transition has been more complete.

oneself as a respectful child in relationship to them. In the secular world, impersonal economic and employment arrangements rather than traditional ties bind one to authority, so such transferential relationships to authority figures could be inappropriate and maladaptive rather than functional.

One consequence of the function of psychotherapy as a means of transition from traditional values is the antagonism of psychotherapy toward religious values inherent in the institutionalization and content of most psychotherapeutic approaches. Institutional practices include the basis against admitting overtly religious people into psychotherapy training programs, the presentation of only non-religious personality theories in texts, the relative prevalence of non-religious people in the mental health professions as compared with their proportion in the general society, the absence of education in psychotherapy programs about the religious beliefs and practices of their future clients, the avoidance of religion as an explicit area of exploration in psychotherapy, and the adherence to reductionistic and clinical views of religious experience (Sollod, 1978a). Such practices argue against the conception of the psychotherapies as neutral, scientifically based forms whose goal is mental health and for a conception that one of the major social functions of the therapies is to facilitate the evolution away from traditional religious practices toward a more secular definition of life.

While there is an appreciation of the role played by religion in other societies and more primitive cultures, American personality theorists and psychotherapists have largely avoided religion and religious motivations as being important subjects of consideration. Murray, who played a seminal role in the development of clinical psychology as a field, avoided listing religious motivations such as salvation, transcendence, and enlightenment in his exhaustive enumeration of human needs (Vitz, 1980). Religious behaviors were included only in a deprecatory fashion. The desire for atonement or confession, for example, was listed under the category of self-abasement. In contrast to his attitude toward religious motives, Murray accorded sexuality and career ambitions a central place.

The selfist orientation of the modern

psychotherapies with their implicitly non-religious focus on the individualized self and its experiences, pleasures and achievements has been viewed as the goal to which contemporary therapy addresses itself (Vitz, 1977). The psychotherapies' view of optimal function-ing is seen as consistent with the assumptions of a modern secular society (Tart, 1975; Bergin, 1980). White (1978) has commented on the fact that the mental health professions equate healthy functioning with a Dionysian rather than Appollonian approach to life. Such an approach would emphasize the benefits of hedonism, impulse expression, creativity, and spon-taneity and would devalue restraint, balance, re-sponsibility, and the patient commitment to long-term goals.

Not only does psychotherapy function generally as an instrument of social transition, but the functions it supports may be quite subtly transmitted and may reflect specific steps in the ongoing evolution of social life. Welkowitz (1978) has provided an in-teresting observation. She noted, in a long-term psychotherapy study, that the attitudes of therapists toward women's roles had changed. At the onset of the study, in 1965, therapists had promoted the roles of housewife and mother. They had interpreted women's career strivings in terms of neurotic conflict. By 1978, the situation was reversed. Women were supported in their expressions of desires for autonomy and pro-fessional achievement whereas their wishes to remain a housewife and mother were often interpreted as in-dications of passivity and lack of differentiation. The recorded nature of actual intervention had also changed with a marked diminution in the frequency with which therapists interrupted their female patients' speech patterns. What was even more striking was that when therapists were asked about their approach to women, they reported that there had been no change. They had, in a prereflective manner, apparently altered their use of psychotherapeutic techniques as a response to general social transition. At both the beginning and end of the study, they had been using psychotherapy to promote a certain type of social adaptation, con-sistent with different views of a healthy woman's role in society. In neither case could their choice of goals be considered obejctive, neutral, or value-free, yet they considered their work to be based on scien-tific theories as well as clinical observations and were unaware of their changing value stances.

A General Model for the Development of Psychotherapeutic Approaches

Based in part on the considerations presented here as well as on studies of psychotherapeutic innovation (Monte, 1977; Sollod, 1978), a general model for the origin and development of psychotherapeutic approaches can be proposed. The innovator of a psychotherapeutic approach may draw from a variety of sources in addition to clinical experience and extant psychological theories. Psychobiographical factors, philosophical systems (Rogers drew quite extensively from Dewey and progressive education), the Zeitgeist, religions, and other disciplines such as education may all play important parts. These factors may also have influenced the innovator's view of reality and may thus be implicit as well as explicitly acknowledged sources of a novel therapeutic approach.

In developing a psychotherapeutic approach, the innovator is often promulgating in a public way a personal solution to those problems posed in his or her own life which had not been resolved through extant social institutions or psychotherapies. In some cases the approach may be seen as a response to problems experienced by patients with whom the innovator has worked. Only close psychobiographical investigations will be able to indicate which, if any, therapeutic approaches have been derived purely from scientific and clinical considerations. One is struck by the fact that in many cases, an approach proclaimed to be derived from such sources actually appears to have become the guiding philosophy of the therapeutic innovator. Wolpe, Ellis, Laing, Rogers, Freud, and Skinner[2] are examples of innovators who apparently based many of their conclusions on clinical evidence, yet clearly believed in the view underlying their therapeutic approach as a guiding philosophy for their own lives. If an approach does gain acceptance and obtains wide adherence, it must have value for people

---

[2]In response to the question posed to him at a symposium at Teachers College in 1979, "What were you before you were a behaviorist?" Skinner replied, "A Presbyterian."

other than the innovator as a means of resolving issues
in their own lives. Thus, a new psychotherapeutic approach may be seen as a solution developed by an individual, often in response to the issues of his or
her life and experience, which has general relevance
to other individuals in society.

Underlying both the general process of therapeutic approaches is the reality of social change. In
its origins, the institution of psychotherapy may be
viewed as a response to the movement from a traditional
religious society to a secularized urban one. It
serves in general as a means of replacing those functions of support, value-maintenance, and socialization
previously provided by the extended family, community,
and religious institutions in a pre-industrial society.
More specifically it facilitates adjustment to the
various steps of a rapidly evolving social world. An
analysis of the social-historical concomitants and an
investigation of the sociological basis of a given approach would provide clues as to the functions fulfilled by a new approach. The skills learned in encounter
groups might come to be seen, for example, as needed
to facilitate a sense of connectedness in an atomized,
impersonal urban world before other institutions such
as neighborhood associations evolved to fulfill the
same functions. Assertive training, in this persepctive, might be seen as required not by a compelling
logic derived from behavioral models of healthy functioning, but by the requirements for survival in a
certain stage of urbanization.

Toward a Reappraisal of the Status of Psychotherapy

In the light of this presentation, psychotherapy
may best be formulated, not as an application of the
science of psychology, but as a group of approaches
and methods which endeavor to facilitate new patterns
of individual behavior and adaptation to society. Such
an endeavor is most legitimately termed an educational
rather than scientific endeavor. Viewed in this way,
the very diversity and lack of organization of the institution of psychotherapy may be considered advan-
tageous as it enables psychotherapy to be flexibly sensitive to the nuances of social change and to innovate
diverse approaches in response to the impact of such
change on individuals. Psychological theories are one
important source of psychotherapeutic innovation,

but--as is the case in other forms of education--a variety of other considerations play a legitimate role. Such considerations may include the values, needs, and aspirations of individuals and the functions society expects from them.

A view of the psychotherapies as a collection of educational forms would be sympathetic to therapeutic innovation but would be more concerned with the motives, directions, and consequences of therapeutic approaches than with the issue of scientific validity. The issues of what philosophies inform psychotherapeutic approaches, the values inherent in them, and the consequences for individuals and society of a given approach would be more openly addressed than would be the case if psychotherapy continues to be examined within a scientific framework. Furthermore, the existence of contradictory psychotherapeutic approaches would be more suitable to an educational rather than scientific framework, where it continues to be somewhat of an embarrassment. The institutionalization of the psychotherapies as educational forms would provide them with significant, though more modest, prestige and yet would strip them of unwarranted claims to scientific authority. The public could become more aware of the limitations and values inherent in various psychotherapeutic approaches. Psychotherapy could still maintain sufficient institutional status to maintain and develop new forms, to provide training for new practitioners, and to maintain a dialogue with other groups in the academic and scientific communities. Finally, the extra-psychological and extra-scientific underpinnings of psychotherapeutic approaches could be acknowledged without seeming to undermine the psychotherapeutic endeavor.

NOTES TOWARD THE HISTORY OF AN ILLUSION

Jacob Needleman

Lately, psychotherapy seems to be moving with great speed in two opposing directions away from Freudianism. The one direction is an attempt to find a more "rigorous" natural-scientific basis for curing patients. Chemotherapy and what has been called "behavior therapy" are clear examples of this tendency. In the other direction we find many schools of thought going under the name of "existentialist," "phenomenological," "humanistic," etc. which in varying degrees reject natural science in the study of man, or relegate it to a secondary status. Certainly, these two tendencies are signs of a growing dissatisfaction with psychoanalysis. Indeed, it seems to some that psychoanalysis has become one of the constellation of individual and collective "pathogenic" forces of which it purports to be the cure, that it is a symptom of a problem rather than a way of resolution.

But of course the interesting question is whether these alternate directions, which we can roughly label Scientism and Humanism, represent a fundamental improvement over the supposed shortcomings of psychoanalysis. The movements which may be grouped under the term Scientism are clearly vulnerable to the charge of over-reductionism. For example, the attempt simply to correlate behavior patterns with physiochemical changes might seem to be conceptually a relatively neutral undertaking. Yet the recognition and description of "behavior patterns" is itself based on certain presuppositions, certain principles of selection which may naively beg the question as to the nature of psychological phenomena. How much more, then, is taken for granted when the Scientist begins by separating "pathological" and "normal" behavior! Rarely, if at all, does the Scientist consider, let alone justify, the value-judgments that may be an essential part of his presumably "objective" description of behavior. I argue that all concepts of pathology, especially of psychopathology, are predominantly valuational. If this is so, the Scientist will have to bring forth a scientific demonstration of the existence of the objective correlates of his value concepts. But since natural science, as I have tried to show, is based on the elimination of value from its encountered universe, this effort is doomed.

To this the Scientist, particularly the behavior
therapist, has an interesting reply: his tecniques
work; patients get better. And they do so incom-
parably faster than by means of psychotherapy. The
behavior therapist understands his task to be the use
of conditioning techniques for the removal of neurotic
and psychotic symptoms. As behaviorist and positivist,
he refuses to acknowledge that there is an entity,
called a "disease," that underlies these symptoms; for
him the symptoms are the disease. Since the symptoms
are forms of behavior, and since all behavior is learned, or conditioned, response, his task is clear: when
a patient comes to him and complains of a symptom, such
as homosexuality or a phobia, the therapist conditions
the symptom away.

    It does seem that, seen this way, the behavior
therapist is simply the purveyor of a technical service, much like a tailor, or, to recall a Socratic
example, a cosmetician. For if one thinks of therapy
as a method of producing health, then it is certainly
a dubious procedure to allow the patient to dictate
to the therapist the treatment of his ailment. It is
precisely because there is a discrepancy between what
bothers me, as a patient, and what may really be wrong
with me that it is necessary for there to exist such
a thing as therapy, either somatic or psychological.
It is one thing for me to go to a doctor and complain
about a pain in the abdomen; it is quite another to
enter his office and request that he remove my gall
bladder. Just as it is one thing for a physician to
perform the service of enlarging a woman's breasts with
silicone injections so that she will feel more attractive to men, so it is quite another for him to refuse
this task and to warn the patient of those physiological ramifications which he knows about much better than
she. So regarded, the various techniques classified
as "behavior therapy" might be more appropriately
termed "behavioral cosmetics."

    In a way, there is a certain appealing frankness
and clarity in such a discipline. If a patient is a-
fraid of cats and doesn't like to be afraid of cats,
she can go to the behavior therapist to have the fear
"removed" much as she might go to the cosmetic surgeon
to have her breasts enlarged. It goes without saying,
however, that the behavior therapist does not think of
himself in quite this way. He speaks of "disorders",

"neurosis," "psychopathology ," and so forth, his
standard of pathology being what he calls "maladaptive
behavior." But I think there are few concepts more
problematic than this.

Obviously, to think of behavior as adaptive or
maladaptive is to treat it as instrumental toward the
realization of an end. But how is the goal or end to
be known? For surely, there are levels of instrumen-
tality; that is, there are goals which are themselves
instrumental for further ends. And, of course, the
immediate goal of a particular pattern of "adaptive"
behavior may itself be "maladaptive" with respect to a
more fundamental goal, etc., etc. In addition, therefore, behavior therapy on its very own terms is obliged
to consider the well-known problem of adaptation to a
"sick society," that is, it raises the ethically and
psychologically formidable issue of "the well-adjusted
stormtrooper." And of course, it must also consider
on an individual basis the "adaptability" of the patient's relatively fundamental life-goals.

Any refusal, under the banner of a positivistic
rejection of the "unverifiable," to scrutinize these
more fundamental goals would be to lapse again, though
more subtly, into cosmetics. Thus, the very project
of therapy should force the behavior therapist to
question in the most serious way the often careless
equating of what is desired with what is desirable. If
he does not do this he ought to change his title to
cosmetician.

In the space of this brief and general essay, we
must pass by many other relevant issues. But in the
light of the preceding discussion there emerges one
point of utmost importance to what is presented as a
phenomenological delineation of "mental illness". The
fact that behavior therapy "works" so well points to
the possibility that all human behavior, all aspects
of our personality, are acquired by a mechanical conditioning process. Indeed, this is the core of the
contemporary theory of learning upon which the techniques of behavior therapy are based. Thus, the
"success" of behavior therapy points, though perhaps
unwittingly, to at least a partial confirmation of
the idea that the distinction between psychic health
and illness must be based upon the mechanicalness of
human behavior. (Naturally, behavior therapy in

substituting one mechanical pattern for another--and in a mechanical way--contributes, in this sense, absolutely nothing toward the patient's health.)

Furthermore, if--as various experiments in learning theory and hypnosis seem to suggest--human behavior, including patterns of thought and feeling, is the result of mechanical conditioning processes, and if psychic health is measured by the degree of freedom from this mechanicalness, then it follows that the organization of human life, as we know it, is essentially pathological and pathogenic.

It has been argued that the failure of Scientism seriously to engage the question of the nature of health and illness is a result of a reductionism in which all entities, including man, are described, i.e. perceived, as essentially the non-vital, non-purposeful materiality of the Cartesian res extensa. Simply stated, the general issue is how to understand man as a part of nature. I believe that some of the enormous difficulty of this problem becomes visible when we see how, in its own way, the humanistic, existentialist reaction to Freudianism also fails to offer a realistic understanding of human nature, its potentialities and limitations.

The Humanist therapist sees man as inherently free, spontaneous, creative and loving. He sees psychopathology as that in the individual which impedes the expression of these elements. His mode of treatment is, fundamentally, to relate to the patient in such a manner as to bring forth this expression--that is, to relate to the patient in a free, spontaneous, creative and loving way. So formulated, the Humanistic psychotherapeutic enterprise seems founded on the assumption that the therapist is healthy, i.e. free, creative, etc.--at least much more so than the patient. That is, psychotherapy is here based on the therapist's faith in his own powers. How does he know he is free, creative, etc.? I think the final answer is that he feels that way. And what he tries to bring his patient to is also this feeling of freedom. In this context, the Humanist complains of Scientism's underestimation and devaluation of man, whereas he claims to have faith in human beings, and to see the positive and strong side of his patients as well as their negative side.

To my mind the critical issue here is not the possible vagueness of such concepts as freedom, creativity and so forth, but the fact that the Humanist denies that these elements can ever be known in any exact fashion. That is, the mode of apprehending them is totally at variance with the mode of apprehending and obtaining knowledge of nature. Not only is it totally at variance, but it must always be so by the very nature of the case. Thus is the order of human experience seen as utterly severed from the order of nature. Behind this severance is the metaphysical postulate of a radical separation between man and nature.

The irony of this position is that it occurs within a general trend of thought which violently disputes the Cartesian dualism of mind and matter and what is called the subject-object split. In fact, however, Humanism remains in essence Cartesian because fundamentally it never questions the Cartesian concept of nature, however much it criticizes the Cartesian concept of the self. Thus, contemporary natural science still remains credited with the only reliable knowledge of nature, and thus nature is still seen as inherently non-vital and non-purposive. Man, being conscious, is thus an ontologically unique specimen who, roughly speaking, stands over against the world of nature. This is so even if his consciousness is spoken of as a relational reality. That is, the power of relating, living, purposing, is still his alone. Nature remains blind, non-relational, non-intentional.

If the knowledge of self is to such a degree cut off from the knowledge of nature, the knower can never be interested in the possibility of external forces that may influence him, or perhaps determine him. He relies on his own feelings about himself because, essentially, he sees no meaningful external corrective to them. And so the idea of development or movement toward a better personal existence, or health, becomes linked to an active striving to feel better either by doing certain things or by relating to other people in certain ways. Thus the therapist's faith in himself and in his patients is based on a trust in the Cartesian estimation of the material world and the unjustified assumption that this is the only sort of nature that could exist. What he feels in himself

61

seems totally different from that nature, and so he
becomes, in this special sense, a law unto himself. At
the best he may speak of a dualism of I-thou and I-it,
but it is a dualism in which nature as an object can
have no influence on his subjective sense of relationship.

But if the Cartesian view of nature is seriously
put to question, and if nature is seen as being itself
organic and purposeful with man one sort of purposing
entity among others, then my knowledge of self depends
more on a search for the way nature influences me than
on an attempt to exercise powers whose general natural
function I do not yet understand and which I may not
even possess. From the perspective of an organic view
of nature, Humanistic psychotherapy becomes another
example of cosmetics, because from such a persepctive
the feeling of power must be distinguished from the
actual possession of it.

If, in some sense or other, I am not the only sort
of entity which can love, if this "power" of loving or
creating or willing, etc. is not ontologically unique,
then my capacity to feel is not ontologically unique
either. This implies that it can be the effect of
something external to myself, and that it can include
an illusional element. That is, if thoughts and ideas
and feelings are part of nature then they are not a
law unto themselves, but have to be approached as
effects at least as much as they can be considered to
legislate our activity.

All of these quite general remarks taken together
with a more detailed criticism of psychoanalysis itself may very tentatively suggest the possibility that
the history of psychology and psychiatry during the
last hundred years is the history of an illusion.
Phenomenology's role in revealing that illusion is to
suggest that our perception and description of the self
is conditioned by our conception of nature (or
"reality"), and that this conception, in turn, cannot
be justified by the scientific method which is based
on it since all the objects which the scientist at-
tends to will be perceived and described in its light.

The illusion of the "pragmatic" criterion is, for
its part, based on several unexamined assumptions about
the job we wish done by our scientific concepts. These

assumptions are, first, that the purposes our conceptual schemes are designed to serve are congruent with
the essentially real, and second, that these purposes
or desires are relatively uninfluenced and unchanged
by that reality.

The first assumption, or hope, can result in our
being satisfied with a theory simply because it
"works", without our questioning those human purposes
which it "works" for--that is, it may be that we do
not, in a sense, ask enough of nature (and our
thought), and thus we bar outselves from the discovery
of our ignorance. An ultimate consequence of this
first assumption may also be the idea that the universe
is non-purposive simply because it does not manifest
the kind and scale of purpose which we would like it
to have.

The second assumption behind the pragmatic
criterion, namely that our purposes and desires are
uninfluenced by "external reality", can block us from
considering the possibility that our general and particular ideas of what knowledge is may themselves be
an effect of natural forces which we do not, in some
larger sense, understand.

Though these illusions are not peculiar to
psychiatry and psychology they are compounded there by
the fact that the pragmatic criterion is not ultimately applied to a reality external to the mind, so that
even the restricted practical success of the physical
sciences is unobtainable. When, in addition, the
idea of health and illness is brought into the picture,
the enterprise becomes almost ludicrous, being the
attempt to ascertain the purpose of non-purposing
phenomena, and, once this impossible aim is reached, to
assist the organism to function optimally in a universe
where the very idea of optimal function has no ultimate
objective correlate. As for the Humanistic trend, we
have seen that it does not deny the metaphysics of
natural science, but merely seeks to make no use of it,
equating the feeling of freedom with the fact of freedom and thereby indirectly supporting what is essentially a Cartesian separation of consciousness and
nature.

The recent growth of interest in religion, particularly Eastern religion, might suggest that a

healthy questioning of modern, Western presuppositions is beginning to take place. Many therapists and theoreticians have attempted in one way or another to make use of Zen Buddhism, for example, or Indian philosophy, or various yoga and meditation techniques. Others, staying more within the Judeo-Christian fold, seek to integrate such religious concepts as atonement, sin, faith and salvation, etc. with concepts pertaining to mental health and illness and the process of psychotherapy. Still others, of course, cite Junigian theories along similar lines.

One of the central ideas of many Eastern religions concerns the ultimately illusory nature of the world men normally live in. This doctrine, as far as I can judge, was not meant to apply only to those we call psychotics or neurotics, but includes--indeed stresses --the illusory nature of the world and life of so-called "normal" man. And so from the persepctive of these teachings the psychiatric distinction between the healthy and the ill appears to dwindle to a very secondary status. Futhermore, this doctrine does not seem to pertain to all entities in the world with the exception of psychotherapists and their concepts, but very much pertains to the reality of the therapist himself.

Thus, for a psychotherapist to take seriously this doctirne of Maya it would be necessary for him genuinely to consider the possibility that everything he bases his thought upon is in error, that every purpose he wishes his thought and action to serve (including the ideal of "helping" people) is a deception, and that he himself, without special guidance and difficult work, must remain a mirage of many colors and little substance which imagines it is a man. That is, the doctrine of Maya, if not taken to apply directly to the inquirer himself, ultimately becomes but another deception. This, of course, is the great embarrassment of genuinely religious ideas: they are meant to be taken personally.

A very similar state of affairs exists with respect to Judaic and Christian ideas. To take only one example, the proscription against idolatry in Judaism and the concept of the poverty of spirit in Christianity both, in their own way, seem to suggest that

64

the movement toward human transformation can begin
only as a man can turn some part of himself away from
the imaginings of strictly human thought, feeling and
action. That is, help comes from God and not from
man, not even from such men as Freud or Heidegger.
The Judaic "broken heart" and the Christian "despair"
which are understood as the precondition of the religious search do seem worlds apart from the psychotherapist's confidence in his judgment as to what in a
religion can be selected out to serve a humanly defined goal of "mental health"--not to mention the confidence he has in his, or his school's, ability to
help his fellows. In any event, we ought certainly
to question whether a genuinely religious idea can be
used to serve aims put forth by men who do not themselves properly suffer the application of these ideas
to their own lives and thought.

It is clear to me that the various new trends in
psychotherapy, though they may be directed away from
psychoanalysis, are still movements in the same plane
and dimension. That is, they are all, directly or
indirectly, intentionally or unwittingly, children of
the modern natural-scientific metaphysics. As such,
they must endure the criticism of the school of
phenomenology, a criticism which requires of them a
drastic re-evaluation not only of their mode of explanation, but of their very perception of the phenomena they seek to explain. Of course, whether
phenomenology in any of its forms can itself provide
a reliable basis for the understanding of consciousness is quite another question. Perhaps, despite all
appearances to the contrary, modern man has not yet
learned how to hear the ancient question: "What is
man?"

PHILOSOPHY AND PSYCHOTHERAPY

PHILOSOPHY AND PSYCHOTHERAPY

The healing profession is, according to Aristotle, properly included under the category of the natural arts along with farming and education. Though each depends to some extent upon principles derived from science they are arts nonetheless for their objective is not mere theoretical understanding but practical results. They are said to be natural rather than creative in the fact that they do not of themselves produce their ends. Rather, through their knowledge of nature they bring together those conditions through and from which their ends will come about "naturally."

This view of the healing professions as natural arts has important implications concerning the current debate among contemporary health care philosophies in general. Its implications for the status and practice of contemporary psychotherapy however, are particularly important. The relation between a natural art and its respective "science" is such that the state of the art depends to a high degree on the state of its related science. Thus, in the biomedical area, for example, the state of the art in medicine is highly dependent on our understanding of the workings of nature in the area of biology. In other words, though an art and not a science itself, the sophisticated achievements of contemporary medicine are due in large part to a correspondingly high degree of unanimity and sophistication in our knowledge of biology. Unfortunately, this is not the situation in the discipline upon which psychotherapy depends, that is, psychology.

There can be no denying that there has been considerable advancement in psychology. Behavioral, developmental and experimental psychology have each made impressive strides in advancing our knowledge of human behavior. Yet notwithstanding these achievements, the discipline of psychology still seems to lack the paradigmatic coherence, method and shared sense of common direction characteristic of the natural sciences. In fact, there are scientists who, all protestations from psychologists to the contrary, simply deny that psychology is a science at all. Their verdict may be supportable by more than merely prejudicial professional arrogance.

Aristotle was not only careful to distinguish the

natural arts from the creative, and the arts in general from their respective sciences, he also distinguished the basic kinds of science from one another according to their object of study. Very generally, the basic kinds of science can be described as 1) those which have as their object the behavior of empiricially observable phenomena (the natural sciences), 2) those which have as their object the laws of logic and mathematics (the rational sciences) and finally, 3) that "science" which has as its object the first principles of the other two and of science itself (first philosophy or "metaphysics"). For Aristotle, a first principle presupposed by every science and of science itself and one which is therefore the proper object of study for "first philosophy" is <u>psyche</u>'.

According to Aristotle, psychology is both and neither natural science and metaphysics. Inasmuch as the study of observable behavior is concerned, psychology may be considered a natural science yet to the extent that explaining and understanding that behavior requires appeal to <u>psyche</u>' as its cause, then it is metaphysical. This may explain the motivation of those "psychologists" who repudiate psychology's more traditional concern with <u>psyche</u>' in favor of exclusive focus on "behavior" in the hope of rendering psychology purely scientific. If they were honest to their origins, however, such exclusively behavioristic orientations might be justified in calling themselves "behaviorology" but they do not properly deserve the title "psychology". True psychology is inextricably rooted in philosophy, not science.

Though the science of behaviorology is essential to the practice of psychotherapy, so too is the discipline of psychology i.e., the philosophical quest to understand ourselves as the source of our behavior—the principles and dynamics of psyche'. True psychotherapy requires not only, nor perhaps even primarily, the ability to change behaviors; it requires an understanding of the basic nature and workings of that for which by definition the therapy is designed—the psyche'. Thus, it is an essentially philosophical enterprise relying as much if not more upon the insights of philosophy as science.

Though science is not completely value neutral in its own presuppositions, the study of values <u>per se</u>

is not the object of science. It is, however, the
object of philosophy. And, inasmuch as the practice
of psychotherapy unavoidably involves appeal to the
analysis of value, it is, as a practical art, as much
dependent upon philosophy for its basis as medicine
is upon biology. A psychotherapy that fails to
acknowledge its essential relation to philosophy but
pretends to be purely "scientific" and value free is
in reality deceiving itself and its clients; it is
simply philosophically and ethically irresponsible.

Questions of value are not the only issues of
uniquely philosophical importance to the foundations
of psychotherapy. There are in addition some basic
conceptual issues whose resolution must be presupposed,
consciously or not, in formulating a psychotherapeutic
model. One of these is perhaps the most basic philosophical question of all, at least it is one of the
oldest. It is the problem of "the one and the many"--
how the question of the relation of unity in diversity
is to be resolved upon which our most basic concepts
of reality depend. Our first essay of this section
addresses itself to precisely this issue as it relates
to the practice of psychotherapy. Though offering a
suggested "resolution" to the issue, it is included
here more to raise our level of awareness of the importance of this philosophical question to psychotherapy than to answer it.

Similarily, the second essay of the section
focuses on a conceptual issue of equal philosophical
importance to psychotherapy--the image of man. Here
our author traces conceptions of the human image in
various psychotherapeutic models and focuses on the
dynamic emergence of this image in psychotherapy, both
in its history as a profession and in its clinical en-
counters. Taken together these essays represent an
initial response to the demand of the previous section
for a philosophical re-evaluation of the nature of man
and his relation to the fullness of being. Again,
their inclusion here is intended to stimulate the
opening of these issues to a more conscientiously
philosophical re-examination than to close them by
providing their "solutions."

The last two essays of the section deal with
psychotherapy's philosophical origins in Freudian
psychoanalysis and the role of philosophy in some of
the more popular contemporary psychotherapeutic models.

The first attempts to demonstrate the essentially,
though not acknowledged, philosophical origins of
psychotherapy despite its pretended "scientific" be-
ginnings. The second analyzes the philosophical world
views of five major therapeutic models and the extent
to which a "cure" under those models depends upon the
client's adoption of, or conversion to that world view.
Taken together these essays respond to the issue of
the "scientific" verses philosophical and educational
aspects of psychotherapy raised in the first section.

PSYCHOTHERAPY: BEING ONE AND BEING MANY*

Charles E. Scott

My purpose is to interpret a fundamental aspect
of therapy by attending to one of the central distinctions in Western thought: it may be called the
part-whole distinction, the problem of the one and
the many, or the issue of identity and difference. The
distinction reflects a pervasive and experienced dimension of human awareness: that in being who I am in
particular I am in my awareness beyond my particularity
in common with all. I shall interpret this situation
by focusing on how we occur in common. That <u>how</u> is a
particular event that reflects non-particular commonality. I shall assume that the coming forth of beings,
how things are available with us, is the place to look
for a thematic understanding of how we are in common,
i.e., I do not view form or matter or subjectivity as
the key for understanding how we are in common. Hence,
the experience fundamental for the part-whole distinction, not its various theoretical formulations, is
my linkage with my great philosophical predecessors.
And the meaning of that experience is our linkage together now as we, philosophers, psychologists, and
therapists, work on an interpretation of the basis of
psychotherapy. We shall be doing phenomenology as we
examine the experiential occurrence of one and many:
our aim is a descriptive interpretation of a central
aspect of human awareness.

1. Theory and Therapy

The relation of theory and therapeutic practice
is seldom clear. When a philosopher speaks about
therapy, the therapist is inclined, intuitively in the
present cultural climate, to hear abstraction and intellectual exercise. And philosophers are inclined to
discount as unsophisticated those ideas developed by
non-philosophical therapists. Experiences, however,
may link theory and practice. We practice out of basic
experiences, and we think out of basic experiences.
When, for example, the categories fundamental for our
thinking have to do for the most part with explanation,
with causes and results, we speak out of a desire for
intellectual order and out of projects related primarily to conceptual structuring. Those desires and
interests mean that thinking in an explanatory manner

*Reprinted by permission of the Editor, <u>Review of
Existential Psychology and Psychiatry</u>, Vol. 16, 1978-79,
pp. 81-94.

is separated from therapeutic practice in which people attend to meanings and events in terms of fundamental affections and affective relations. At least that appears to be the situation presently in that the meanings of affection and the meanings of explanation are usually ordered in highly different ways. But if the thinker and the therapist find common experiences to think out of and use discipline in attending to these common experiences, an accord of theory and practice can occur. In that accord, thinking enriches and guides practice and practice guides and enriches thinking. Our interpretative aim should be to find and attend to common events and to relate and speak out of those specific instances of commonness.

When we attend to our commonality and see that commonality in relation to therapeutic events, therapeutic practice and thought regarding therapy will reflect each other in an area of growing awareness that is made up at once of theory and practice. That awareness is our aim, and it is not attainable as a thought or as an object of thought. Rather, this kind of awareness comes as one listens to the events and experiences out of which this discussion arises and which are reflected in the discussion. As concepts reflect and speak of events common for us, our awareness develops. Then we may say that interpretation, in the sense of growth of understanding and development of common meanings, is going on.

2.   Plato, Parmenides, and Heraclitus

There is a relation between unity and order that has been experienced as not efficiently caused. Order is found not to be done by any particular direction of will. The Greek experience of destiny is an instance. Directions are ordained by the fabric of possibilities, nature, and particular human beings. Like the inexorable moving of a suspended wheel, like the seasonal course of the heavens, situations move toward fulfillment of directions, toward intrinsic completion, without regard for specific human interests or personal fulfillment. Destiny is a self-completing unfolding of situation or setting that is not defined by its many participants. This notion of destiny has spoken out of people's awareness that the whole of the situation of which they are a part is not deeply informed by the strength and charcter of individual passion.

That whole may be thought of as the Cosmos all around a located human being, or it may be thought of as the non-personal dimension of human being. In either case, the person is deeply and sometimes terribly aware of an infinitely transcending region which is regardless of the individual's fulfillments and suffering. My emphasis presently is to fall on how this non-personal and non-volitional region has been found and how it is significant for understanding our own well-being.

I want to note, without developing further, how Plato, Parmenides and Heraclitus spoke of the immanent presence of a region which transcends individuals, which is in some sense comprehensible, and which is present as a direction of non-personal unfolding in personal experience.

Plato speaks of the intimate and intrinsic link of unchanging beings to changing beings by saying that the unchanging "becomes in" the changing being or is "to be in," "to lie in" the changing being. The non-personal "comes to be" in the individual's circumstances. A particular finite being is "in common with" its defining, but transcending reality. They are "in communion with each other," and the finite being "imitates" or "is like" its present and transcending destiny as it lives out and toward what is given to be.

The defining reality of a given thing is not the specific, existing thing, but is its order, its particular unity. This unity is found to be different from the vicissitudes of the existing thing, but definitive of what the thing, in spite of itself, can be and become. It is an instance of destiny. And for Plato, unity means goodness. The unfolding of a being's destiny, its definitive reality, is a reflection of the unity and wholeness that enjoys sway over everything. I understand that to mean that Plato discovered that the present non-personal directions of his being, when thoroughly included in the individuality of his own way of seeing, inspired a fulfilling completeness that was good in its occurrence.

This experiential correlation between well-being and non-personal unity is also reflected in Heraclitus' and Parmenides' fragments. Heraclitus combines a method of reflection that "distinguishes each thing according to its own way of being" with an encompassing insight that "what is common to all," how we are in common, can guide us. Guides us in what sense? "Nature loves to hide," he says and is not usually available for direct knowledge. Things, however, find their "repose in changing," and "conflict" and "strife" provide direct access to the repose in common of all things. Such claims are paradoxical only if we view all things solely from the perspective of individuality. How we are in common guides us in how change occurs. The measure of kindling and dying down, waxing and waning, victory and defeat and so forth is defined by none of its instances. Again we find the insight that order is an event of relation between individuals and non-individual aegis, a relation susceptible to sight, but not to explanation. The meaning of this aegis is found by Heraclitus in that soul that lives out its "inner law" to fulfillment as a "dry beam of light." Seeing for Heraclitus, as it is for Plato and Parmenides, is an occurrence in which one gives way to the seen and does not interfere with how it is. Only then can human awareness undergo an ordering in which it finds its partiality to reflect thoroughly that unity or wholeness which defines awareness without being that awareness.

"Gaze steadfastly," said Parmenides, "at things which, though far away, are yet present to your mind. For you cannot cut off being from being; it does not scatter itself unto a universe and then reunify." He found being to be one, common and utterly the same in all of its instances. This sameness is utterly compelling when seen, only and simply as it is; it is that without which differences could not occur; it is present always and always not an instance of anything. The intensity of Parmenides' experience of the meaning of the sameness of being should not be overlooked: the scattered is always in common and reposed in its being; the scattered is not to be denied, but the common repose is to be intimately known.

Plato, Heraclitus, and Parmenides each know that order is found in a present non-object which need not will to be and which in its presence makes possible an accord among the many that need not overcome differences, strife, and relative agreements in order to be at one and deeply at peace.

3. Difference and Diversity

76

We experience difference and diversity in terms
of puzzlement, privacy, opposition, resistence, identity, and self-differentiation. The child discovers
that he/she is not the same as his/her mother. The
adolescent discovers he/she is not the same as his/her
father. The adult discovers that he/she is not the
same as life itself or being itself, i.e. he/she
discovers that he/she is to die. We all discover that
we are different from the world of which we are intimate parts, and I believe that puzzlement accompanies
these discoveries. One may not think about the discovery. He/she may not ever know that the discovery
is going on. He/she may simply see his/her mother or
father or him/herself differently. He/she may feel
pause or doubtful or set apart. He/she may laugh
or fall quiet in his/her puzzlement, but an experience
of question occurs as such transitions occur. The
words odd or remarkable or strange would probably be
appropriate for such experiences. I suspect that most
of us at one time or another wish, out of our puzzlement, that we were more at one with things such that
doubt and question were not so pervasively appropriate.

In the puzzle of being different, we are immediately aware of ourselves in our silence, in what we do
not say, in how no one absolutely knows us, in our
capacity to say yes and no. We occur as private in our
differences. As private we are opposed. We can experience the "no" of others, their privacy, their
differences, their refusal of us or of our intentions.
And we have a sense of who we are in our difference
and privacy. We are name and identity to ourselves
in our being different with others.

But the most problematic experience presently
appears to be self-differentiation rather than differentiation with others. We tend to think of ourselves
exclusively in terms of our specific identities with
others, which means not only that a backdrop of loneliness is particularly characteristic of our present
manner of being together, but also that we expect to
be just exactly who we are. I take this literalism of
identity to be expressed in resistance to one's dream-
ing awareness, in remarkable conceptual stress on the
ideas of personality and character when one wishes to
understand human reality, in the identification of consciousness and conceptual mentality, and so forth.
When we occur to ourselves as significantly different
from the way we usually are, we may be surprised,

shocked or traumatized. If I am this one identity, private and different from everyone else, how can I possibly also be different from myself? How can I be mother and father to myself? How can I be my own shadow. How can I desire what I abhor?

I shall indicate later that this kind of literalism is lived as a refusal of one's sameness, of one's own being. Presently I want to stress that difference from everything else but oneself and difference from oneself are aspects of how we are in common. Consequently, doubt, question, puzzlement, and a thorough absence of sameness are given aspects of our world and of ourselves in our particular being.

4. Indifference

Difference, as distinct to indifference, occurs by virtue of immediate interest and concern. As I feel desire things distinguish themselves, and as desires change, foci and penumbra change. I am a region that is alert in desires and interests. I am aware of myself in relations marked by intricate and familiar networks of interests, commitments, concerns, i.e. networks of desires. Desires are living, aware directions which have the power of singling out and ignoring and which give energy in some relations while letting other relations fall out of importance.

As a person I am a self-aware region of desires. That region is subject to changes in the hierarchy of interests, to shifts in relations, satisfactions, failures, and so forth. But I am immediately aware of myself in desiring, in being interested, in seeking, avoiding, finding, struggling, etc. Differentiating in concrete relations is at the core of personality and character.

As I differentiate in desiring, I find all manner of things tat are not what I am after. Intense desires are particularly powerful ways to distinguish things. Hatreds and loves, as we know so well, set things apart and bring things together, discover sames and not-sames, and give fundamental identities to things in their desiring contexts.

Not desiring at all might well seem like death to us, at least the death of our identifiable selves, our

78

individuality, our character. Our being particular, that is, our specific way of being just who we are, occurs in distinguishing things. Our identity is intimately involved in the manyness of beings. In our desiring we find the world highly diverse, potentially fulfilling and threatening, filled with beings that come and go and change always.

Indifference has a puzzling quality about it. By indifference I do not have in mind ignoring something or someone. Ignoring is an attitude. I have in mind an absence of attitude. This absence of attitude is seen in the notions of one and whole. The whole context of all our many situations is not attitudinal or personal. What Heraclitus, Parmenides, and Plato knew, viz. that indifference is always an accompaniment of differentiation, that indifference is never resolvable into differentiation, that the one is not the many--that knowledge was partially recovered some years ago when nature ceased being viewed through the metaphor of mother and, after some initial, heated disappointment, was allowed to be impersonal, indifferent, and yet beautiful. I say partially recovered because we have yet to appropriate fully in our contemporary setting the fact that indifference is the horizon of all differentiation. The nursing mother, for example, who provided so much meaning for people's experience of nature, is not only personally and uniquely related with her child. She is also mother. It is child. Feeding is occuring. The very quality of eternity which we might experience in the nursing situation is beyond all the individual caring and specific nurturing that is going on. The metaphor of mother nature can mean that mother is pervaded by indifference even as she particularizes and gives individual nurturance.

This absence of attitudes is a dimension of human awareness. It is constitutive of the world as we live it. A pervading sameness, a non-differentiated, non-individual unthing-like quality may be found with all instances of things. It is a non-caring, non-desiring, non-differentiating dimension that we are sensitive to when we know, for example, that we die without regard for our interests, that we change regardless of how we change, that meaning occurs in spite of what meanings there are, that being is regardless of our desires, that personality and character occur no matter what their content.

Indifference names one aspect of how reality is.
It is important for our interests because it also
names one way in which what has been called the one,
the same, or the whole appears. Therapeutically indifference is important because it not only names a
dimension of our own existence which can be terrifying,
but it also names the wholeness of our being which can
be refused or blocked only with enormous expense to
our being well.

If we absolutize the personal for psychotherapy
either in our language or method, we shall leave out
of account the very being of our existence, that is,
the event or the coming forth of things, in such a
way that plurality and individualism will be limits
for our understanding of health. Desire, in that case,
would appear to be the foundation of human existence,
and all experiences would be lost in which desire steps
back of impersonal insight, uncaring contemplation,
aimless intuition, and desire-free communion. Our refusal of indifference means insensitivity regarding
not only nature in its difference from us, but also the
very quality of seeing the undesired or the totally un-
expected, as frequently happens in insight. Such refusal means that our appreciation for the non-personal,
such as I-Thou occurrences, would be seriously
damaged. It would also mean that we would tend to
identify knowledge of objects with awareness as such.
Indifference names the non-objective, non-particular,
non-desiring dimension of our awareness, the immediacy
of awareness, in which no person is found and on which
personal well-being is founded.

5. An Instance of Part/Whole: Awareness of Meaning
and Awareness of Meaning and Awareness of Meanings

By looking at our sense of meaning in relation to
our senses of meanings we shall take one example of
the simultaneity of particular and whole, and that will
give us at least some orientation toward understanding
the meaning of our being at once one and many. My aim
is to direct us toward an interpretation of human being
in which we can see that oneness is a fundamental event,
not an accomplishment, and that as that event is lived
in denial it is accompanied by psychological illness.

I want to focus on how meanings reflect the sheer
event of meaning, how a meaning is a phenomenon of an

event of which the particular meaning is a part. "Participate" won't do to speak of this relation of part-whole, because that notion tends to mean two separate things which are characterized by one thing's being in the other thing. We would have thereby begun with a primordial separation of realities which means that the whole would be taken as an entirety of the parts. The basic words which I shall use to name the part-whole presence are _event_ or _occur_. The advantage is that these two words may say how we are aware of whole and part without meaning that part and whole are separated things.

Whole is not experienced as a thing or as a part of a larger context of experience. When Heraclitus, for example, spoke of Logos as the unity of all change I do not think he had reference to an entity posited by intelligent guesswork or to a particular thing in his experience. He addressed by his notion of Logos a non-objective awareness of sameness, a wholeness which happens as diversity happens.

This starting point is significant for us here insofar as we want to understand how therapy happens with two or more persons. We might speak of our sharing common properties or of our participating in common process or of our privately enjoying experiences that are similar. But such manners of understanding assume from the outset a separateness that takes no account of being same together in its point of departure. Such accounts make wholeness either something to be accomplished or to be found from a particular perspective. Particulars are not received, from the beginning, as phenomena of sameness when we speak of participating in a common process, privately enjoying similar experiences, or sharing common properties. In such instances, we give a virtually unchangeable primacy to particular perspective.

But meanings precede perspectives in a linear as well as in a founding sense. When we speak as though particular perspectives are primary for either meaning or awareness, we misstate in a deeply forgetful way the primacy of meaning with respect to all particular points of view.

A point of view is always a meaningful part of a meaning event. Shall we say that that event of meaning is like a body of water that contains a particular drop of water which we note particularly? Meaning is not like a body that holds and contains. Meaning is an event of relatedness that allows for identification. Things are already together in certain ways such that we may occur in particular ways regarding them. Our regard, our awareness in our particular manner, is our being related in certain ways with things that are already together with us in certain non-perspective ways.

'Existential analysts' such as Bingwanger have located the general characteristics of human experience in the a priori structure of human experience. We, however, are following those who locate such aspects in the 'world', that is in the identifiable relatedness of things and not in an a priori structure of mind or experience. And we are noting that world-relations themselves constitute our awareness as the foundation of our perspectives. How things are together and how we are with them is the region of awareness, as distinct to a posited, interior brain structure. Further, the wholeness or the sameness of the event of many fluctuating particulars is to be found in the already together quality of the event itself. Things being apparent in their own relatedness is the region for inquiry when we want to understand our experiences of part-whole.

Meaning names an occurrence that tolerates an apparently immeasurable range of differences. Things are good, bad, indifferent, threatening, inviting, or whatever. But in any case they are present as something: they are nameable and related. Meaning seems to be an horizon that cannot be totally transcended, even in radical experiences of meaninglessness, since these experiences are founded in nameable world-relations which are experienced as disconnected or falling apart. Meaning, though not like a physical container, is pervasive, an immeasurable sameness that tolerates an infinite range of differences and opposites. And human awareness occurs as meaning event: it is at once a situation free of the individual, and individual stance in that situation, and a pervasive occurrence of meaning regardless of the contents of the meanings.

We may consequently speak of an awareness of

meaning as well as of awarenesses of certain meanings.
One is always found with the other, but neither is the
same as the other. An awareness of meaning happens
indifferently vis-a-vis which meanings occur, and
that awareness is defined without regard to which desires, interests, comedies, or tragedies are going on.
And yet, without an awareness of meaning as such,
the world would be totally absent, i.e., 'we' would
have no sense of relatedness, identity, or particularity.

6. Metaphors for the Experiences of The Whole

Metaphors for the experiences of the whole are
frequently ones of depth or of light; down deep, un-
derneath, back behind, feelings of depth and descent,
translucent, pervasive shades, light of lights, like
the light of the sun, and so forth. Metaphors of
hearing could be used just as well, if not better; pervasive sound, backdrop of silence, unsounding harmony.
In any case, pervasiveness and distance without objectivity are important aspects of the meaning of the
experiences of the whole.

'Whole' is being one's own event. We are never
finally circumscribed by any one particular situation
or by any one set of factors which identify us particularly. Being whole is, as classically seen,
transcendence of that particularity which is also real.
Parmenides doubted the reality of particularity and,
closely related to Parmenides' doubts, Plato doubted
the reality of change and changing things. None of
us can share these doubts now, in the way they seemed
unavoidable to Plato and Parmenides. We are more inclined to doubt whatever casts relativity on change
and on a presumed absoluteness of particularity. We
are more inclined to doubt the whole of being our own
event than we are to doubt the idea that change is
absolute.

In our classic, metaphysical tradition the reality
of the whole or the one tended to be identified as a
permanent kind of thing. The very notion of the whole
may connote a circumscribed being which is all that
and none of this: identical with itself. We must dis-
associate, however, the idea of the whole from the
context of permanent and changing things if we are to
be attuned to the experiences of wholeness. It does

not occur as something permanent or as something changing. It does not occur as a thing at all. We experience the whole as an alertness that pervades and casts an horizon vis-a-vis all present things. We could call it non-voluntary readiness for experience in the midst of experiences, awareness that pervades opposites, a sense of the limitedness of identity, the mood of finiteness, alertness that goes beyond and beneath all that I reflect and know, a sense of sameness with all the differences of my experience. It is like light that illumines all lighted things as far as one can see. It is like darkness that cannot be grasped or seen through: dark into dark. It is like a tone reaching the limits of audibility and seeming not even to stop there. It is like a silence that is heard with sounds. It is like an unfathomable and unreachable source that is as it is, but does nothing in particular.

7. When I Am Afraid of the Eventfulness of My Being

My relation with my own eventfulness, my own being, always involves a sense of the limitedness of who I am in particular. When I identify my being with my particular way of going about things by crystallizing myself into patterns that I take to be absolute for me, the eventfulness of my being will be deeply and inevitably threatening at every level of my particular awarenesses. My self-understanding will need to be protected. What I possess will need to be guarded and defended. Ownership will foreshadow repeated crises of danger and attack. My sense of place will need constant reinforcement to make clear its fortification against change. Peace will seem to be the opposite of open freedom. Definition will need the enforcement of strong commitments. Fixity will need guarantee. Guarantee will need defense. My very eventfulness will be a constant taunt of the particularities of my life. My life might feel deeply and vaguely decayed, like there is something gnawing at the core. Death might feel like a hand taking away something precious. The horizons might seem like boundaries under imminent attack. The danger of loss, defeat, and perhaps poverty will pervade my successes, fulfillments, and affective riches. I will be utterly at odds with my own being.

When I am at odds with my being in that way, and

when I am with you, I will be inclined to attack or
defend or hide or control. But I will not be inclined
to be together with you in the horizons of awareness
where who I am in particular fades back of our being
together. I will immediately and non-reflectively
define our relation in terms of interests and intentions. I will want to build or tear down or change
or keep things as they are, that is, I will want to
do something. But I will not seek touch with that
non-particularity of the event of being together which
happens in the aims and interests of our relation, but
which is itself neither aim nor interest.

Being out of touch with my eventfulness, my wholeness, is like bieng out of touch with any other dimension of my own reality in this sense: I cannot feel
close to it even when I focus on it or think about it.
It will seem distant even when I know about it. It
will seem inappropriate or suffocating or emptying in
its closeness. I will seek to protect myself from it,
and in whatever protection I find I will be solidify-
ing an opposition to dimensions of my own being.

When I am opposed to the eventfulness of my own
being I will be predisposed to blocking openness and
pervasiveness at all points in my existence. I will
want to control by bowels as well as my children. I
will feel the threat of merger and loss of identity
in all dimensions of relating with others that do not
involve clarity of intention and a sense of control.
I will want to exercise a maximum jurisdiction over
the details of my death. I will tend to define consciousness in terms of structures of knowledge, and
I will tend to define my psyche in terms of volition.
I will tend to find the meaning of my life solely in
projects and accomplishments. I will find open and
free listening difficult. I will find deep serenity,
as distant to happy relaxation, impossible, and I
will seek, perhaps compulsively, confirmation of the
value of the particulars of my life.

The oppositions which are part of my existence
will, in this situation of refusal, tend to seem un-
natural or wrong or contradictory. If my tendency is
toward moral judgments, I will feel wrong and guilty
to be different from the favorable aspects of my being. If my tendency is toward literalism, I will
tend to deny the existence of my own self-differences.

I will generally think of truth as different from contradiction and opposition, such that I will be un-
prepared to face the enormous range of opposites and
differences that make up being human.

8. When I Welcome the Eventfulness of My Being One
   and Many

I am swaying back and forth among the words oneness, unity, wholeness, and eventfulness because
wholeness, unity, and oneness traditionally have
named the region of pervasive non-diversity. But I
have used event and eventfulness in an effort to set
our thinking apart from the traditional inclination
to attach to wholeness or unity the meanings of either
changelessness or sole claim to being or the characteristic of being a separate thing in relation to other
things. And I have said that wholeness is not an
object of awareness, but is a dimension of awareness
that is immediately and non-personally self-aware. The
eventfulness of human being is the occurrence of
awareness in its pervasive immediacy.

We have seen that this dimension of our occurrence is an experience in the sense that we live it
unavoidably and with non-objective sensibility. It
pervades all aspects of our lives. But we are free
to assume various stances regarding it. Among those
postures, we may reject it or welcome it in all manner
of ways.

Therapeutically, when you address and confirm the
claims of my being, you may need to remain silent
regarding the claims of my personality. My particular
way of being may well be opposed or hostile to how my
being is. I may fear my own occurrence as whole and
non-personal. I may be angry over my own inevitability of change, given my desire to keep what I like.
I may deeply resent and view as evil the inevitability
of my death, given my enjoyment of me and my life. I
may hate the pervasiveness of loss even when loss
means the growth of my children or of a friend or
the maturation of possibilities in a situation which
I liked in its nascence. I may not like being limited,
and I may seek to defy the limits of my being. Or I
may not like the intangible and indeterminate presence
of possibility and seek to eliminate as much inde-
terminancy as possible. If any of these situations

are true of me, and I am your patient, I shall want
you to confirm and support me in my usually non-
conceptualized refusal of my being. I shall want you
to attend to my particular way of being at a distance
from my being. In a word, I shall want you to support
my refusal of my own occurrence. What will you, my
therapist, do? Won't you hear the claims of my being,
the occurrence of deathliness, limitation, possibility,
indeterminacy, intangibility and change? Won't you be
at peace with them and welcome them as you hear me and
my disturbance? Won't you remain silent when I seek
you to confirm me, in order that you may give place and
time for my event, my occurrence as human?

And yet you always address me in my partiality
as you address the claims of my being. I may be
divided against myself in hostility to the claims of
my being. I may be tight and pinched and blocked in
my fear of the claims of my being. I may be so distant from those claims that I dash madly about at times
in which slowness is appropriate and am hardly capable
of movement when speed is most appropriate for the
aims of a given situation. So as I seek your confirmation for the sake of justifying or confirming my way
of being, you, whom I trust, let us say, remain silent.
And yet you admit, allow, and accept me in my particularity. No resistance from you, no denial. In
admitting me freely in our way of being together, you
have allowed me my denial of myself, my hostility or
fear regarding how I occur, or whatever the case may
be. Your non-confirming allowance of my particular
way of being admits at once the claims of my being and
how I am in particular. When depth therapy occurs,
I am freed for my being in acceptance of how I am
denying it.

Perhaps I now overplay the obvious when I say
that in welcoming the eventfulness or wholeness of my
being, I find myself free for diversity, difference
and opposition as characteristic of my own existence
in my being with others. I may now be open to be as I
am in my particularity as well as to be transcedent of
my identity in the very occurrence of my reality. I
occur as part/whole, or -- and I intend to say exactly
the same thing as part/whole -- I occur as an event of
awareness that is in a particular way.

The wholeness of human being is not an achievement,

and when I welcome it I am in that welcome free from
the necessity of validation of my being by means of
accomplishments. The wholeness of human being is not
a specific situation; and when I welcome it, I am
free from the demands, responsibilities, and opportunities which also define my place and position. As
I allow it, i.e., do not resist and refuse it, the
freedom for being whole pervades these demands and
opportunities which also define my place and position.
As I allow it, i.e., do not resist and refuse it, the
freedom for being whole pervades these demands and
opportunities and is lived as my not being enslaved
or destroyed or finally defined by them. I am then
deeply free for change, in those particularities and
consequently in my self-understanding and identity.
The difference of wholeness vis-a-vis particularity is
my freedom in my being from the identity of a particular way of being. This difference may be lived,
for example, as hope when one's life is desperate
or as the capacity to change even when one's life is
happy, or as an uninhibited desire for growth when one
feels generally satisfied with the particulars of his/
her life or as what we name vaguely, but significantly,
soul and the German language names Mut, i.e., that
disposition which is the desire to be as distinct
to the desire to be one thing in particular. I believe
that Freud made reference to this difference made by
freedom for the wholeness of one's being when he spoke
with Binswanger about resistance to therapy. He noted
that there is often a time in therapy when the patient
may turn toward a healing process or away from it, and
that, he said, is a time over which the therapist
has no control. I believe that is a time when one is
faced with the experiential meaning of welcoming or
turning away from the eventful quality of his/her own
being.

I might turn away because I am deeply and pre-
cognitively convinced that I will simply pass away if
I do not affirm absolutely the way that I am alive.
Absorption might be the primary object of my fear. Or
I might be terrified of a total insignificance which
might come if I do not second by second insist upon
my way of being. Welcoming the wholeness of my being
might well feel like opening my arms to dying or like
sinking into a deep sea or flying endlessly and aimless-
ly with no control. These terms are founded in my
immediate awareness of the difference between being
partial and being whole. The positive direction of the

terror is my sense that if I cease being partial in the way in which I now am, I cease to be. The meaning of the pathological direction is my ignorance of wholeness as compatible with intense partiality.

If you are my therapist and seek to respond with my terror in such instances, you will have the difficult task of hearing my being with my particularity. I will need to learn in my relation with you that I can welcome my wholeness without dying or totally losing my sense of myself. Perhaps I will make this non-intellectual discovery as I find myself repeatedly accepted by you in many diverse or opposing ways. Or in your freedom for whatever I am unfree for in myself. Surely there are uncountable ways in which such awareness occurs. But whatever its mode, I shall be able to welcome the wholeness of my being with you only as you and I touch or hear with and behind our words and silences and feelings and aims that occurrence pervasive of all that happens, the wholeness, the occurrence, the happening itself, which is always with, but never the same as what is going on.

When I welcome the happening of my being, its events, I happen with the oneness of existence. I am immediately in touch with the strangeness that there are beings, that this and this and this is. As Parmenides, Heraclitus, and Plato knew, the wonder of things is not found exclusively or even primarily with reference to their idiosyncrasies. Their particularity is necessary in their occurrence, i.e., that's the way these things are, but there is also an occurrence of reality, an event, the very opposite of a vacuum. It is the coming forth of what is there, its being there, not absolute dissolution, but coming out as things; not total darkness, but lighting up; not absence, but being. Welcoming the happening of my being open with this unfixable region of awareness which I have named the wholeness or the event of being. When this welcoming openness is a part of my particular way of being, I suspect that I will no longer need extensive therapy with you.

PSYCHOTHERAPY AND THE HUMAN IMAGE

Maurice Friedman

An important aspect of my three books on the image of the human--Problematic Rebel, To Deny Our Nothingness, and The Hidden Human Image--has been exploring the meeting between the image of the human and psychotherapy. Each school of psychotherapy has, with varying degrees of clarity, its own image of the human. That image stands in fruitful dialectic with the therapeutic practice of the members of the school, but it is not, for all that, a scientific product of that school. On the contrary, the far-reaching differences between the many schools of psychotherapy derive in part from the fact that implied in the positive goals they enunciate are different images of the human. Such central therapeutic terms as "health," "integration," "maturity," "creativity," and "self-realization" not only imply an image of the human, but also usually essentially different ones for different schools and even different members of the same school. "The critical battles between approaches to psychology and psychoanalysis in our culture in the next decades, as always," writes Rollo May, "will be on the battle ground of the image of man." (Friedman, 1964)

Human nature is often taken by schools of psycho-therapy to be itself the norm. The human being should live according to his "nature," according to his "real self," and the like. However it is also a part of human nature to become ill. The very meaning of "health," therefore, implies some sense of what is authentic direction for the human being, for this particular person--in short, an image of the human. As Helen Merrell Lynd points out, the "real" or "spontaneous" self is not a given that need only be freed from its social encrustations. It is the pro-duct of a lifelong dialogue with our image of the human.

Horney, Fromm, and even Sullivan at times, seem to assume that there is an already existent real or true or spontaneous self which can evoke into active existence almost at will. There is a tacit assumption that somehow we know the dictates of the real self, and that we should

91

live in terms of these rather than of a
romanticized self-image or of the pseudo-self
of others' expectations. But. . . such a real
self is something to be discovered and created,
not a given, but a lifelong endeavor. (Lynd,
1969, p. 203

Especially helpful in Helen Merrell Lynd's On
Shame and the Search for Identity are her clear insights into the implications of various personality
theories for the image of the human which a particular
psychology or psychoanalytic theory assumes, and her
recognition that such images are matters of basic
assumption even more than of scientific evidence and
methodology.

It does make a difference whether the individual is considered as eager, curious, and
trusting until specific experience in a given
society and historical period lead him to be
anxious, cautious, and aggressive, and fear which
specific experiences may modify only to a limited
degree in the direction of trust, sympathy, and
interest. (Lynd, 1969, p. 142).

The possibility of mutual relations "between
persons as an enlargement, not a contradiction of individual freedom," is incompatible with personality
theories "that see men primarily as need-satisfying
objects or in terms of their particular status or role
relations to oneself" quite as much as with those
theories center in "release of tension, return to
quiescence, and self-preservation." "Much depends"
she writes, "upon whether one believes that isolation
and alienation are inevitable in man's fate or that
openness of communication between persons, mutual
discovery, and love are actual possibilities."

On the basis of the "death instinct" which he
ranges alongside the "love instinct" as equally primary in Civilization and Its Discontents Sigmund Freud
presents a devastating image of the human which no
person who lives in the world today can afford to
ignore:

Not merely is the stranger on the whole not
worthy of love, but to be honest, I must confess
he has more claim to my hostility, even to my
hatred. He does not seem to have the least

trace of love for me, does not show me the slightest consideration. If it will do him any good, he has no hesitation in injuring me, never even asking himself whether the amount of advantage he gains by it bears any proportion to the amount of wrong done to me. What is more, he does not even need to get an advantage from it; if he can merely get a little pleasure out of it, he thinks nothing of jeering at me, insulting me, slandering me, showing his power over me; and the more secure he feels himself, or the more helpless I am, with so much more certainty can I expect this behavior from him towards me . . . .

The bit of truth behind all this--one so eagerly denied--is that men are not gentle, friendly creatures wishing for love, who simply defend themselves if they are attacked, but that <u>a powerful measure of desire for aggression has to be reckoned as a part of their instinctual endowment</u>. The result is that their neighbour is to them not only a possible helper or sexual object, but also a temptation to them to gratify their aggressiveness on him, to exploit his capacity for work without recompense, to use him sexually without his consent, to seize his possessions, to humiliate him, to cause him pain, to torture and to kill him. (Freud, 1958, pp. 59-61)

<u>Homo homini lupus</u>, Frued concludes: Man is a wolf to man. "Who has the courage to dispute it in the face of all the evidence in his own life and in history?"

Who indeed? In the years since Freud's death in 1939 there has been as much new evidence of "man's inhumanity to man" as in the whole of recorded history up till that time: the Nazi extermination of six million Jews and a million gypsies, the bombing of German cities, the atomic destruction of Hiroshima and Nagasaki, the slave-labor campus of the Soviet Union, the wars and uprisings and systematic exterminations. The view of man as an essentially good, rational creature who will gladly co-operate with others in his own self-interest is no longer a live option. Such evidence cannot be excluded from any serious contemporary image of the human.

It is evidence, nonetheless, of how man <u>acts</u> and

93

not of what man is. Like the myths that Freud uses, it is a plausible, perhaps even a convincing hypothesis, but one that can never be scientifically verified. Since we cannot know either instinct or human nature outside a historical context, we cannot categorically assert, as Freud has, that the desire for aggression is a part of man's instinctual nature. It would be equally possible to say with Erich Fromm that the destructiveness which human beings vent on one another is the product of an authoritarian character structure which is, in turn, the product of one or another type of authoritarian society. What is not possible is to ignore the enormous amount of hostility and destructiveness that human beings have displayed toward one another in history and in our own day. Rousseau held that man is by nature good and that it is only civilization that makes him bad. Freud, with much greater realism, recognizes that civilization is inseparable from man. In this sense, it is meaningless to ask what man is "by nature," since we only know him as a social and civilized being. For the same reason, it is not necessary or even possible to accept Freud's view of "human nature" at face value. But it is necessary to confront his view of the human with utter seriousness and to take it into our own, hopefully large, human image.

Jung criticizes Frued for seeing man as basically evil, and he himself characterizes the "evil" side of the self as the "shadow," the complement of the good. If it is not suppressed, this "evil" can be brought as such into that very integration which Jung calls the "self," thus achieving a type of wholeness in which the individual knowingly succumbs to evil "in part." Good and evil are both relativized here to mere functions of wholeness. Human values are transcended by "the voice of nature, the all-sustainer and all-destroyer." "If she appears inveterately evil to us," says Jung, "this is mainly due to the old truth that the good is always the enemy of the better." But what is this "better" of which he speaks? It is that "individuation," or wholeness in the unconscious, which has no reference, check, or court other than itself, no direction, guide, or criterion by which to distinguish one voice of the archetypal unconscious from another. If we still recognize apparent evil in the unconscious, then it is our task, for the sake of

this "better," to succumb to it in part so that we
may realize our destiny:

> The inner voice brings the evil before us
> in a very tempting and convincing way in order
> to make us succumb. If we do not partially
> succumb, nothing of this apparent evil enters
> into us, and no regeneration or healing can take
> place. (I say "apparent," though this may sound
> too optimistic.) If we succumb completely, then
> the contents expressed by the inner voice act as
> so many devils, and a catastrophe ensues. But
> if we can succumb only in part, and if by self-
> assertion the ego can save itself from being
> completely swallowed, then it can assimilate
> the voice, and we realize that the evil was,
> after all, only a semblance of evil, but in
> reality a bringer of healing and illumination.
> (Jung, 1954, p. 185)

What sort of "healing and illumination" does
this "semblance of evil" bring? Jung's immediate
answer is that "the inner voice is a 'Lucifer' in
the strictest and most unequivocal sense of the word,
and it faces people with ultimate moral decisions
without which they can never achieve full consciousness and become personalities." But Jung's concept
of a "moral decision" is very different from the old
distinctions between right and wrong, just as the
court of conscience is replaced for him by the
criterion of wholeness and the address of the inner
voice. If the healing that such "moral decision"
leads to is not obvious, still less is the "illumination" it provides: "The highest and the lowest,
the best and the vilest, the truest and the most
deceptive things," reads the very next sentence,
"are often blended together in the inner voice in
the most baffling way, thus opening up in us an abyss
of confusion, falsehood, and despair?" What is the
way out of "this confusion, falsehood, and despair?"
It is succumbing in part to evil, or, as Jung puts
it in a later writing, not succumbing to either good
or evil, but rising above them, which means, once
again to relativize them. The Carpocratian Gnostic
teaching of going along with one's own body in its
instinctive demands is cited favorably by Jung in
Psychology and Religion and is freely read by him
into Taoism as what must, according to his own insights, be the secret of Taoist detachment:

Have we, perhaps, an inkling that a mental attitude which can direct the glance inward to that extent owes its detachment from the world to the fact that those men have so completely fulfilled the instinctive demands of their natures that little or nothing prevents them from perceiving the invisible essence of the world? Can it be, perhaps, that the condition of such knowledge is freedom from those desires, ambitions, and passions, which bind us to the visible world, and must not this freedom result from the intelligence fulfillment of instinctive demands, rather than from a pre-mature repression, or one growing out of fear? (Jung, 1931, p. 80)

In his critique of Jung in Eclipse of God Buber confesses that he is particularly concerned by Jung's Modern Gnostic resumption, under the guise of psycho-therapy, of the Carpocratian motif of mystically deifying the instincts instead of hallowing them in faith. "The soul which is integrated in the Self as the unification in an all-encompassing wholeness of the opposities, especially of the opposites good and evil, dispenses with the conscience as the court which distinguishes and decides between the right and the wrong. It itself arbitrates an adjustment be-tween the principles." This "narrow as a knife's edge" way leads Jung to the positive function of evil when it is integrated in the "bridal unification of opposite halves" in the soul which is the goal of the process of individuation. The self which is in-distinguishable in its totality from a divine image and the self-realization which Jung describes as "the incarnation of God" goes back, Buber points out, "a Gnostic figure, which probably is to be traced back ultimately to the ancient Iranian divinity Zurvan (not mentioned, so far as I know, among Jung's numerous references to the history of religions) as that out of which the light god and his dark counter-part arose. (Buber, 1957, p. 86-90, 136f).

Erich Fromm criticizes Freud for seeing man as anti-social by nature and only secondarily in re-lationship, whereas Fromm holds, as does Harry Stack Sullivan, that man becomes destructive only when his neurosis turns him aside from a creative relationship with other people and with his work. For Fromm, human nature is potentially good or evil, with health on the side of good. It is significant, however, that Fromm was not content with his explanation of the evil of Nazism as the product of authoritarian society and character structure in <u>Escape</u> <u>from</u> <u>Freedom</u> and went on to ever deeper and more extensive analyses of human evil in <u>The Heart of Man</u> and his voluminous study <u>The Anatomy of Destructiveness</u>.

In <u>The Heart of Man</u>, in probably conscious response to those who have accused him of ignoring the repressed negative aspects discovered by depth psychology, Fromm discusses "the most vicious and dangerous form of human orientation." This is the love of death, malignant narcissism, and symbiotic-incestuous fixation, three orientations which combine in their extreme form into a "syndrome of decay" that prompts destruction and hate for their own sake. In opposition to the necrophilous person, Fromm posits a "biophilic <u>ethics</u>" which is clearly his own image of the human:

> Good is all that serves life; evil is all that serves death. Good is reverence for life, all that enhances life, growth, unfolding. Evil is all that stifles life, narrows it down, cuts it into pieces. Joy is virtuous and sadness is sinful. . . . The conscience of the biophilous person is not one of forcing oneself to refrain from evil and do good. It is not the super-ego described by Freud, which is a strict taskmaster, employing sadism against oneself for the sake of virtue. The biophilous conscience is motivated by its attraction to life and joy; the moral effort consists in strengthening the life-loving side in oneself. (Fromm, 1964, p. 47)

Attractive as this emphasis is, it does not bring us appreciably closer to a direction-giving image of the human than the "productive orientation" of Fromm's <u>Man for Himself</u>, to which Fromm himself refers. Not even the status which Fromm gives this image by his claim that "the pure biophile is saintly" can rescue it from the fatal ambiguity of what is meant by "life." Fromm cannot capture the human in the sheer love of life since the human being's relation to life is different from that of the rest of life. Life is not worth loving and enjoying unless implicit in the concept of life is living well.

Growth is not necessarily a good unless implicit in
the concept of growth is growth in a direction that
realizes positive values. Fromm's syndrome of growth
does indeed imply such values--love, independence,
openness--but for that very reason his scheme is
circular. His ethics of growth rests on another set
of ethics which in turn he seeks to ground in the
ethics of growth.

In Man for Himself Fromm recognizes that what
man is cannot be understood without including what
man ought to be. "It is impossible to understand him
and his emotional and mental disturbances without
understanding the nature of value and moral conflicts."
Yet he defines the source of values in purely pragmatic terms, the good being what contributes to the
mature and integrated personality, vice being what
destroys it.

> The character structure of the mature and
> integrated personality, the productive char-
> acter, constitutes the source and the basis
> of "virtue." . . . "Vice," in the last analysis,
> is indifference to one's own self and self-
> mutilation. Not self-renunciation nor selfish-
> ness but self-love, not the negation of the in-
> dividual but the affirmation of his truly human
> self, are the supreme values of humanistic
> ethics. If man is to have confidence in values,
> he must know himself and the capacity of his
> nature for goodness and productiveness. (Fromm,
> 1947, p. 7)

Fromm presents us here with a succession of terms to
each of which we have a positive emotional response--
"mature," "integrated," "productive," "affirmation
of his truly human self"--but to none has he given
concrete content. He defines values in terms of
"the mature and integrated personality" and "the
truly human self," yet these terms themselves imply
values and would have to be defined in terms of values.
Thus, Fromm offers us one set of explicit, conscious
values which are merely instrumental and another of
implicit, assumed values the source of which he does
not explore. Fromm bifucates "conscience" into an
authoritarian conscience that demands submission
out of fear--not too different from Freud's conception
of the conscience as the introjection of the censure
of the father--and a humanistic conscience which is

"the guardian of our integrity." The humanistic
conscience "is the voice of our true selves which
summons us back to ourselves, to live productively,
to develop fully and harmoniously--that is to become
what we potentially are." But what is meant by the
"true self" and by becoming what we potentially
are?" Fromm knows the beneficial results of authentic
existence, but he cannot point to such existence itself. Thus he falls into the trap of psychologism,
self-realization, and aiming at the self.

For the American psychologist Carl R. Rogers, in
contrast to Freud, Jung, and Fromm, human nature is
unqualifiedly good. Roger's theory of the complete
acceptance of the "client" by the therapist is based
on the assumption that the client is "good" in his
depths, that he is by nature social and constructive,
that all he needs is to be accepted by the therapist
so that he may accept himself and he will make manifest the socially good person that he really is.
Martin Buber's reply to Rogers on this point suggests
that there is a third alternative to seeing man as
"evil," to be controlled, or "good," to be trusted,
and that is seeing him as "polar" and in need of
personal direction: "What you say may be trusted, I
would say stands in polar relation to what can least
be trusted in this man. . . . The poles are not good
and evil, but rather yes and no, acceptance and
refusal." (Buber, 1965, p. 179)

"The aim of therapy is often that of helping
the person to be better adjusted to existing circumstances," says Fromm in Beyond the Chains of Illusion:

> Mental health is often considered to be nothing
> but this adjustment, or to put it differently,
> a state of mind in which one's individual un-
> happiness is reduced to the level of the general
> unhappiness. The real problem . . . need not
> even be touched in this type of psychoanalysis."
> (Fromm, 1962)

"Psychologists and psychoanalysts," writes Helen Lynd,
"have given more encouragement to the adjustment of
individuals to the realities of a given society than
to personal differentiation and deviation from them."

> They frequently fail to give explicit recognition
> to the distinction between normal or healthy

in terms of what are the generally accepted
norms of the society and in terms of what is
humanly desirable. If the psychoanalyst. . .
does not rigorously examine his own values in
relation to those of society, he almost inevitably tends to accept tacitly the dominant
values of the society as the norm of behavior,
and to measure health and illness by these.
Scientific objectivity, then, becomes indistinguishable from social determinants. (Lynd,
1969, p. 212)

Even if the psychoanalyst does rigorously re-
examine his values, as Lynd suggests, he is still
likely to impose them under the mask of objectivity;
for he is not going to lose his values through
examining them. It is true, as Fromm says in Man for
Himself, that it matters whether the therapist encourages his patient to adapt or strengthens him in
his unwillingness to compromise his integrity. It is
also true, as other therapists would point out, that
the patient is sometimes so tied up in his neurotic
rebellion against the culture that there is little
else that he could do anyway. In either case, the
therapist cannot take the risk of encouraging the
patient to oppose society and to undergo privation unless he has a sure enough sense of that perons in his
uniqueness. He must feel sure that the client has a
ground on which to stand as a person and that he
stands there in some real and creative relationship
to the society that he is going to oppose. Otherwise
the therapist cannot help encouraging a patient to
adjust to this particular society and seeing his
health and sickness in terms of that adjustment.

In Beyond the Chains of Illusion Erich Fromm
tells how he began at first with the "strictly orthodox Freudian procedure of analyzing a patient while
sitting behind him and listening to his associations."
This procedure turned the patient into the object of
a laboratory experiment, says Fromm. He was able to
fit the patient's dreams into his theoretical expectations, but he was still talking about the patient
rather than to him. Eventually, he found a new way:
"Instead of being an observer, I had to become a participant; to be engaged with the patient; from center
to center, rather than from periphery to periphery."
That this means an even more radical departure from
the traditional method than Harry Stack Sullivan's

"participant observer" is suggested by Fromm's remark to me that he not only sees therapy as "healing through meeting" but that he believes that the therapist himself is healed in the process. This stress on participation does not mean that Fromm is under an illusion about therapy being fully mutual. Even while he felt himself fully engaged, as he had never been before, and learned that he could understand his patient rather than interpret what he said, he discovered that he could at the same time remain fully objective--seeing the patient as he is, and not as Fromm might want him to be. "To be objective is only possible if one does not want anything for oneself, neither the patient's admiration, nor his submission, nor even his 'cure.'" The therapy takes place for the sake of the cure, but a genuine wish to help protect the therapist from being hurt in his self-esteem when the patient does not improve or being elated about "his" achievement when he gets well.

The image of the human has more to do with therapy itself than it does with our theories about therapy, important as the theories may be; for there is always the danger of the theory becoming a construct in which the therapist settles down. "Young therapists often regard the dreams of their patients as examinations," Fromm said to me. "They feel that they must be ready to give some theoretical interpretations, and as a result they do not really hear the dreams." When he was working with thirty of us in Washington, D.C., in a series of seminars on dreams and the unconscious, Martin Buber said that there are two kinds of relationships a therapist has to dream--one in which he puts them into the categories of his school and the other in which he responds to them spontaneously and wholly in a "musical, floating relationship." "I am for the latter," said Bubber. This musical relationship in which the therapist really hears the unique person and experiences his side of the relationship is crucial for all therapy, regardless of the school or theory. No matter what school the therapist comes from and no matter what knowledge and experience he has, the basic question is still <u>when</u> his insights apply to this particular patient and when not. To answer this question he must use the categories of his school in a flexible, "musical" way in order again and again

to try to arrive at this person's uniqueness. To do
this the therapist must practice what Buber calls the
act of "inclusion," experiencing the patient's side
of the relationship as well as his own. Rollo May
stresses the centrality of such inclusion for therapy
and love in terms of what might be called a "field
theory" of the emotions:

> Our feelings, like the artist's paints and brush,
> are ways of communicating and sharing something
> meaningful from us to the world. Our feelings
> not only take into consideration the other person
> but are in a real sense partially formed by the
> feelings of the other person present. We feel
> in magnetic field. A sensitive person learns,
> often without being conscious of doing so, to
> pick up the feelings of the persons around him,
> as a violin string resonates to the vibrations
> of every other musical string in the room. . . .
> Every successful lover knows this by "instinct."
> It is an essential--if not the essential--
> quality of the good therapist. (May, 1969, p. 91)

Even the patient's "sickness" is part of his
uniqueness; for even his sickness tells of the road
he has not gone and has to go. If instead the
therapist makes the patient into an object to himself,
as well as to the therapist, he will have robbed him
of part of his human potentiality and growth. This is
not a question of a choice between the scientific
generalization and the concrete individual, but of
which   direction is the primary one. Is the individual regarded as a collection of symptoms to
be enregistered in the categories of a particular
school or are the theories of the school regarded as
primarily a means of returning again and again to the
understanding of this unique person and his or her
relationship with his or her therapist? An increasingly important trend in psychotherapy suggests that
the basic direction of movement should be toward the
concrete person and his uniqueness and not toward
subsuming the patient's symptoms under theoretical
categories or adjusting him to some socially derived
view of the "ideal" man. This trend emphasizes the
image of the human as opposed to the construct of the
human. The image of the human retains the understanding of the human being in his or her concrete uniqueness; it retains the wholeness of the person. Only a

psychotherapy which begins with the concrete existence of the person, with his or her wholeness and uniqueness, and with the healing that takes place through the meeting of therapist and client will point us toward the image of the human. In the last analysis the issue that faces all the schools of psychotherapy is whether the starting point of therapy is to be found in the analytical category or the unique person--in the construct or the image of the human.

The revelation of the human image--its coming forth from its hiding--is a revelation that takes place between the therapist and his or her client or among the members of a group. It cannot be equated with the image of the human that each holds or comes to hold separately. The coming into the light of the hidden human image is inseparable from the dialogue itself---a dialogue of mutual contact, trust, and shared humanity. In this sense "healing through meeting" is identical with the revelation of the hidden human image. It is a becoming of the human in relationship--becoming human with such resources as the relationship affords, including the possibility of tragedy when such resources are lacking. It is not the diploma on the wall which assures the client that he has the right therapist. The "rightness" of the relationship depends upon mutual existential trust--and upon an existential grace that is not in the therapist or in the client but moves between the two.

SIGMUND FREUD AND THE QUESTION OF HUMAN AGENCY

Joseph F. Rychlak

One of the more fascinating aspects of studying Freud is the constrasting interpretations which arise as we try to characterize this great theoretician as either a biological reductionist hence physical determinist, or, as a teleologist relying upon a unique form of psychic determinism. I hold to the latter position, and would like in the present chapter to document my views by discussing his relations with four colleagues--all of whom confronted Freud on the question of human agency in one way or another. I will then conclude the chapter with a few observations on the salutary role which philosophical analysis might have played in the evolution of psychoanalysis, had Freud only been more inclined to employ it.

Freud's Confrontation with the Telic Mind

In 1845, eleven years before Freud's birth, four aspiring physiologists studying with Johannes Müller at Berlin, formed a pact to "fight vitalism" in their future scientific careers (Boring, 1950, p. 708). Vitalism in physiology referred to the Galenic view that living organisms were energized by unobservable forces which mixed with the ebb and flow of blood to stimulate life and nourish the body. The four men who dedicated themselves to battle vitalism were Carl Ludwig, Emil du Bois-Reymond, Hermann von Helmholtz, and ErnstBrücke. Some 35 years later, the last of these individuals mentioned found himself a leading figure in physiology, holding a professorship at the University of Vienna. Ernst Brücke was at the top of his career, and no one thought more highly of him than an eager young medical student, who actually dallied three years beyond the date at which his medical class graduated because he hoped to enter academia working under his beloved professor of physiology (Jones, 1953, p. 53). This eager young medical student was Sigmund Freud.

Galenic vitalism mixed theology with medicine, seeking to rationalize a "Divine Plan" in the creation and manifestation of life. Intentions, reasons, or the "ends" for the sake of which God created life are wound into this account of how it is that the human body supposedly functions. The Greek word for end is telos and hence theoretical accounts of this sort are referred to as teleologies or telic descriptions. Teleologies borrow from the meanings of final causation or, "that (reason, grounds, plan, purpose, intention, etc.) for the sake of which things exist or events are being carried forward. The patterned "that" being put into effect in final causation is termed a formal cause--as in the example of God's "Divine Plan." It is possible to have more than one form of teleology. Galenic medicine encompasses a deity teleology, but we can have a human teleology without thereby assuming that a deity is directing events. It is also possible to have natural teleologies in which no assumption is made about a Divine Plan directing things toward some intended or "pre-determined" end.

Even so, what Brücke taught Freud about scientific descriptions amounted to a blanket dismissal of all forms of telic description. If it appears that there are "ends" toward which biological events are moving, said Brücke, the natural scientist must work a bit harder to find the underlying causes of these apparent final causes. Traditionally, in natural-science accounts, this involved a so-called reduction to the material- and efficient-causes substrate which presumably enters into the constitution of all observed patterns (formal causes) and/or purposive outcomes (final causes) (see Rychlak, 1977, Chapter 1).

Brücke's preferred reduction was to the energic forces at play due to the principle of constancy. This principle was introduced by Julius Robert Mayer but greatly popularized as the conservation-of-energy principle by Brücke's fellow pact-member, Hermann von Helmholtz. The principle of constancy says that in any isolated (or, closed) system, the sum of forces at play remain constant--i.e., seek a uniform level of distribution--so that if there is a mobilization of forces at one point there is an immediate and automatic mechanism brought into play which reduces this disparity in pressure points and re-establishes the balance. Helmholtz's refinement is to say that mobilized energy points may be found in such items as wood or coal, which when burned release "so much" heat to boil "so much" water and release "so much" steam, and so on. In a completely closed system the level of potential energy ("so much") would remain constant

106

though it can change its form. This change may appear directed, it may give the impression that events are heading toward some end, but this is merely an illusion based upon an unscientific assessment of what is taking place. The forces of nature are neither divinely inspired nor directed. These forces move blindly along, based upon relative pressure points in the total distribution of energy (efficient causes) or potential energy ("Matter" or material causes).

Freud's dream of becoming Brücke's assistant never materialized, but the professor did help the student obtain a small traveling grant to study in Paris during the year 1885. It was here that Freud came under the influence of Jean Charcot, a famous pathological anatomist who rivaled Brücke in distinction. As Wittels (1924) later pointed out, Freud found in Charcot someone who "maintained, and could prove (in his hypnotic experiments on hysterics), that mere ideas were able to cause disease. It is probable that Freud was not slow to realize that he was learning something which would bring him into collision with the Viennese School" (p.31). On his return to Vienna from France, following a brief stay in Berlin, Freud enlivened an association he had begun years earlier with Josef Breuer. Breuer, in turn, introduced Freud to Wilhelm Fliess so that by 1887 we have some of the first letters of the Freud/Fliess correspondence being drafted. Whether or not Freud was quick to recognize what the French were teaching him about the possible causes of mental illness we cannot say (he later visited Bernheim as well), but the relations with Breuer and Fliess both were to end in the conflict between traditional, reductive, natural-science description and a new style of explanation which took into consideration the patient's mental ideas and treated them seriously in the style of the French.

The professional tie with Breuer ended first. The Breuer-Freud (1955) Studies on Hysteria appeared in preliminary-communication form in 1893, but it is fasinating to note that in 1892, left to himself, Freud proposed an explanation of neurosis entirely at the level of ideas. I refer to his paper entitled "A Case of Successful Treatment by Hypnotism" (Freud, 1966a), in which Freud employed the constructs of a counter-will and antithetic ideas to account for hysterical disorders. This--Freud's very first!--theory suggested that human beings both intended to act in certain ways

107

and yet also hold certain expectations concerning the
likelihood that they can actually put these intentions into effect. There is a subjective uncertainty
in behavior, and with many if not all intentions we
human beings immediately think of counter-intentions
as "antithetic ideas" to those intentions we really
want to affirm and thereby reach "motoric action" in
behavior. We think "I will do that" and immediately
the dialetical opposite is suggested "I can't do that."
At certain low points in life, whether through fatigue
or extended conflicts, these antithetic ideas can take
over and manifest themselves in various types of
counter-willed symptoms so that people "do" what they
have no intention of doing. The mother who does not
wish to disturb her child's sleep makes a clacking
noise with her tongue and the child awakens, or the
highly religious person who would not dream of taking
the Lord's name in vain curses uncontrollably.

The fact that Freud thought of these actions as
two lines of willful behavior suggests that he did not
begin from a natural-science base. The principle of
constancy was surely not directing his theoretical
style here. I have argued that he was, in fact, basing
his theory on a dialectical logic rather than on the
unidirectional thrust of a demonstratively conceived
principle of energy expenditure. Had Freud forgotten
his lessons from Brücke on "how to" be a proper natural
scientist? Not at all. But we see some interesting
maneuvers going on in his subsequent development as
theorist, beginning in his relations with Breuer as
they worked on the Studies. It is significant that we
find Breuer (1955) and not Freud including a constancy
explanation in his theory of hysteria (pp. 196-200).
The editors of the Studies cross-reference this Breuer
usage with Freud's concept of neuronic intertia which
he employed in the "Project for a Scientific Psychology," an unfinished work which we will consider in a
moment (see below). My only point here is to stress
that Freud's explanations were not like Breuer's in
the Studies.

Breuer's argument begins by stressing the fact
that all cases of hysteria stem from "an abnormal ex-
citability of the nervous system," whether or not this
stems from a psychic origin (Ibid., p. 191). He goes
on to use a constancy explanation by suggesting that
there is in a human organism an innate "tendency to
keep intracerebral excitation constant" (Ibid., p. 197).

108

If such abnormal excitations are not "abreacted"
hysterical symptoms can result. How does this come
about? In time, Breuer suggests, the "idea" (memory
of the reason why abnormal emotions occurred) becomes
split off from the rest of the psyche and functions at
a subconscious level (Ibid., p. 226). Why does this
splitting take place? Because, suggests Breuer, of
an innate disposition to what he called the hypnoid
state (Ibid., pp. 235-236). Freud, on the other hand,
was presisting in his "will" theory as follows: "I
was repeatedly able to show that the splitting of the
content of consciousness is the result of an act of
will on the part of the patient; that is to say, it is
initiated by an effort of will whose motive can be
specified" (Freud, 1962a, p. 46). This is the fundamental rationale for what Freud then called defence
hysteria and, of course, in time the constructs of
censorship and repression were to develop from this
style of theoretical explanation.

As for the hypnoid state theory, Freud succeeds
in bringing it down through a series of brief theoretical references in papers on related topics. In
1895 he states that though hypnoid hysteria is an
important hypothesis, every hysteric he has treated
has "turned into a defence hysteria" (Freud, 1955,
p. 286). In 1896 he notes that "there are often no
grounds whatever for presupposing the presence of such
hypnoid states" (Freud, 1962b, p. 195). He then adds
that if one only searches deeper into the psyche he
will find a repressed defense in time. This seems a
kind of reverse reductionism, in which moving from
physical symptom appearances we can in time discover
an underlying psychic ramification of the disorder.
Rather than formal/final causes reducing to material/
efficient causes we have the reverse. Finally, in
1908 Freud dismisses the phenomenon of a hypnoid state
as supposedly due to the physiological sensation of a
protracted pause following a climax of intense sexual
release (Freud, 1959, p. 233). As such, it plays no
role in the etiology of neurosis.

What has happened here? It is clear that Freud
is departing from the traditions of medical explanation to suggest that mental disorders are strategized
maneuvers encompassing dialectically clashing intentions. I say "dialectical" because there is a fundamental contradiction going on in the personality
which defends against making conscious or "acting out"

109

what is already known unconsciously. The mind is in
conflict over the ends to be attained or made manifest
in actual or overt behavior. There is a reason
(formal-cause plan, assumption, projected goal, etc.)
for the sake of which (final cause) the person behaves
as he or she does. Freud found this style of ex-
planation--whether gleaned from the French or not--
much to his liking in understanding his clients and
providing them with insight. Wittels (1924) later
noted how the Freudians developed a "love for tri-
partite subdivision" (p. 34) in speaking about the repressed wish, the repressing wish, and the compromise
worked out between them, and so on. This kind of
"mentalistic" explanation undoubtedly struck Freud's
colleagues in medicine as unscientific nonsense, a
return to Galenic vitalism of one sort of another.
Freud's sexuality thesis served a positive role here,
for it took the spotlight off his telic style of
description and made it appear that anyone who opposed
his explanations of neurosis was doing so entirely on
the basis of the threat posed by personal remnants of
an infantile sexual fixation. I do not say that this
was Freud's intent, of course, but surely he was
equally or more vulnerable on this theoretical style
of description as he was on its sexual content.

Freud's struggle with telic description--or, "psychic
determination" as it is usually framed--is even more
evident in his relations with Fliess. Fliess was as
committed to the biological-hereditary reduction as was
Breuer, if not more so. He had a kind of biological-
clock theory, one which held that both men and women
were moved emotionally by periodic cycles of 23 or 28
days. Depending upon critical periods within this
cycle, the person was said to be vulnerable to neurosis.
Ultimately, Fliess' theory as Breuer's hinged upon a
genetic link of some sort making people vulnerable to
what Freud (1954) once called a "weak spot in the
nervous system" (p. 51) or some such--a predilection to
break down in life when stress occurred. Freud gave
credence to Fliess' speculations for a time, and, as
his life-long physician and friend Max Schur (1972) has
noted, Freud even submitted to a personal treatment
based upon Fliess' theories (p. 95).
    Fliess' influence on Freud was immense, both in a
personal sense and also in the strictly professional
relationship which the two men enjoyed. They used to
meet together in some resort city of the area from time

to time, and exchange ideas in what they called
"congresses" of two. In September of 1895 such a congress was held, and we can piece together from the
course of subsequent events that Fliess had in fact
brought home to Freud the need for firming-up his
theory of neurosis with a biological rationale.
On the train, returning home to Vienna, Freud began
writing what is now called his Project for a Scientific
Psychology. By October of 1895 he had completed and
sent off to Fliess three parts of a projected book.
And one month later, in November of 1895, he could say
to Fliess: "I no longer understand the state of mind
in which I concocted the psychology (the Project)"
(Freud, 1954, p. 134). Though Freud was to produce 23
volumes of work, he was never to finish the Project
and years later when Fliess' copy   turned up
Freud tried to have it destroyed (he had long since
burned his own copy). Even so, there are those today
who would argue that the Project is central to Freud's
theoretical preferences.

        I cannot accept this view, but I do find the
Project of great interest because of the opening para-
graph, in which Freud makes it clear that he hopes to
write a psychology of energic changes (called Q) and
containing material particles in the reality of the
neurones (Freud, 1966b, p. 295). This teaches us that
he had not forgotten Brücke's rule on how to write
good, natural science--bring it down to efficient- and
material-causes! But the fact that he could not finish
this conventional account gives mute testimony to the
kind of theoretician Freud was--which is anything but
a biological reductionist (see Rychlak, 1968, Chapter
VII, for a complete discussion of this issue). Freud
was now to have the same collapse in relationship
with Fliess that he had experienced earlier with
Breuer, and for the same reasons. In January of 1896
Freud (1954) writes to Fliess, suggesting that though
Fliess is trying to understand humanity via physiology
he (Freud) "secretly" nurses the hope of arriving at
this same goal through "philosophy" rather than biological reductions (p. 141). Later that year, Freud's
father died (October, 1896) and in the same year
Freud's famous self-analysis began. From this time
forward we see an emphasis on the early years in the
etiological dynamics of neurosis, culminating of course
in the infantile sexuality thesis (Ibid., p. 183). By
May of 1897 Freud has developed his "layers of mind"
conception and the Oedipal conflict is being brought

in as well (Ibid., pp. 202-203). In September of 1897
Fliess learns that phantasies may be the cause of
neurosis, rather than anything "real" which has
happened in the person's past (Ibid., p. 215). Over
the next year Fliess continued to hound Freud for
explanations of an organic nature, so that by September of 1898 we find Freud defensively asserting that
he does not disagree with this theoretical need in
principle: "But, beyond a feeling of conviction (that
there must be such a basis), I have nothing, either
theoretical or therapeutic, to work on, and so I must
behave as if I were confronted by psychological factors
only" (Ibid., p. 264).

The final collapse of the Freud-Fliess relationship occurred in 1900, during one of their congresses
at Achensee. Fliess insisted that periodic processes
were involved in all psychic activity and that Freud
was a mere "thought-reader" who projected his own ideas
onto his clients (Ibid., p. 324). Freud's reaction,
according to Fliess, was to turn the whole affair into
a personal attack of great animosity and violence.
That Freud began "analyzing" Fliess as a demonstration
of the usefulness of his self-proclaimed scientific
method is reflected in the following, which is taken
from one of the last letters Freud sent to his former
friend: "I was sorry to lose my 'only audience,' as
our Nestroy called it. For whom shall I write now? If
as soon as an interpretation of mine makes you feel
uncomfortable you are ready to conclude that the
'thought-reader' perceived nothing in others but merely
projects his own thoughts into them, you really are
no longer my audience, and you must regard the whole
technique as just as worthless as the others do"
(Ibid., p. 337).

The last person I would like to take up in relation to Freud's confrontation with the telic mind
is C.G. Jung, who was an avowed teleologist, heavily
reliant upon a dialectical construct in his theorizing
(see (Rychlak, in press). By looking carefully into
the Freud/Jung letters (McGuire, 1974) we can see an
interesting continuation of Freud's problems in
accounting for human mentation. Freud's theoretical
strategy following his break-up with Fliess was to retain a psuedo-constancy notion in his libido conception.
I say this was a "pseudo" drive theory because the true
source of Freudian dynamics always springs from a
dialectical ploy of some sort, rephrased in energic

112

terms. It was not merely the instinctual drive or its energy which provided action in a straightforward, demonstrative fashion, but the energy as stimulated and the opposed by some other source of energy --with the resultant repression, projection, or sublimation-- that gave the personality description its uniquely Freudian flavor. Freud even admitted that his libido theory derived more from biology than the findings of psychoanalysis per se (Freud, 1957, p. 79).

Even so, both Jung and Freud accepted the seeming requirement to account for mentation by way of some kind of energy. In a letter of December 1910 we find Jung trying to defend the libido construct, which already had come under attack by Alfred Adler (McGuire, 1974, p. 382). Jung tries, over the next several months of 1911 to bring libido into his studies of the zodiac and other mythological motifs (Ibid., pp. 408, 421, 427). The explanations of these conceptions continue to reflect Jung's basic commitment to dialectical oppositionality, and libido for Jung has to fit in here in some way. Jung hopes to bring libido under an oppositional umbrella, relating to both ends of a contradiction, or a negation. However, in November of 1911 Freud nails libido down to a single energic source, as one of at least two basic life drives--i.e., as the "power behind the sexual drive" (Ibid., p. 286). The following month Jung tells Freud that he is trying to conceptualize libido in a global sense, one which transcends the more "recent-sexual libido" in the course of life to base the psyche as a whole on this elan vital (Ibid., p. 471). Freud and Jung's relationship is very strained at this point, and the disagreement over libido is wound into the supposed motives which each man has for agreeing or not agreeing with the other. We are back to that ad hominem aspect of psychoanalysis noted in the attack on Fliess, so precious in the context of self-study but actually harmful in the context of abstract debate. Though Freud considered it an opportunistic move to curry favor with the detractors of psychoanalysis, Jung's so-called dexexualization of libido as a theoretical construct was actually an elevation of the construct in the over-all theory.

In Jung's hands, libido loses its analogical relation to a physical energy. It becomes the desired value of a person's intention, reflecting the worth of a goal for the sake of which the person behaves (Jung, 1961, p. 111). Libido is said to be experienced as conation and desire, very much as in Schopenhauer's concept of Will (Jung, 1964, p. 147). And most important of all, libido is always brought about through a dialectical oppositionality, beginning in the first efforts of mental differentiation and carried on throughout life according to what Jung now calls the principle of opposition. Thus, by the late 1920's we find Jung saying: "I see in all that happens the play of opposites, and derive from this conception my idea of psychic energy" (Jung, 1961, p. 337).

Being fundamentally suspicious of the dialectic (see Rychlak, 1968, p. 323), and still unsure of himself concerning the question of telic behavior, Freud could never quite take the theoretical step which Jung did. In 1912 he publically apologized for using a teleological argument in "guessing the purpose of Nature" (Freud, 1958, p. 247). I think that Freud was a revolutionary thinker in his personality theory, but he remained a transitional figure when it came to questions of scientific protocol. He was courageous in sticking to his intuitive understanding of human behavior, but he also thought of himself as a scientist. Dialectical conceptions and the telic theories they generated were "out" in the science of his day, and reductive explanations were decidedly "in." To his credit, Freud refused to relinquish his insights concerning mind, insights which in fact relied upon dialectical maneuverings and compromises which gave psychoanalysis a clearly telic intonation.

I think that one of the most important summations of mind he ever made occurred in the Psychopathology of Everyday Life, where he beautifully points out how the distinction between conscious and unconscious behavior does not render the question of agency in human behavior meaningless; phrasing things in terms of "free will," Freud (1960) observes:

> According to our analyses it is not necessary to dispute the right to the feeling of conviction of having a free will. If the distinction between conscious and unconscious motivation is taken into account, our feeling of conviction informs us that conscious motivation does not extend to all our motor decisions....But what is thus left free by

114

one side receives its motivation from the other side, from the unconscious; and in this way determination in the physical sphere is still carried out without any gap (p. 254).

Though Freud was prone to speak of the illusion of free will, he meant by this that what one side of the mind claims is a decision freely made--made "free" of the other--is in fact the effect, outcome, compromise, conclusion, implication, wish, and so forth, of the other side of the mind. Freud never says that mind is incapable of making choices, of deciding, or intending to carry out some end. He could not very well say this for his study showed precisely the reverse in every thing that his clients did. His problem was how to "say" mind behaved "for the sake of" such intended ends without thereby offending the traditional Newtonian science within which he was intellectually reared.

Philosophical Analysis and Freudian Theory

Freud's problem as theoretician was obviously not a psychological or even a scientific one. His concerns and the maneuvers he employed to resolve the tensions of his confrontation with the telic mind were clearly along the lines of a philosophical or philosophy-of-science analysis and/or dispute. I have always thought of philosophy as that human endeavor which instructs us concerning what we already "know" by presumption in anything that we seek to understand, believe in, talk about, and so forth. In this sense, the philosopher is like a special type of psychoanalyst, looking behind the "manifest" content of our beliefs, attitudes, hunches, etc., to find there a "latent" content which necessarily influences the overt meanings under conscious extension. Despite his avowed interest in philosophy, Freud (1954, p. 162) was not fond of technical philosophical analyses per se. He objected to the phenomenological approach which Mach was taking to physics, and yet this is precisely the kind of philosophical approach which he could have used in preference to the reductive libidinal alternative which he actually selected (see Rieff, 1959, p. 26).

Clearly, what psychoanalysis needed at its inception was a firm philosophical base, one which would contrast it unequivocably with the Lockean-Newtonian traditions of 19th century science. Freud was surely intellectually equal to the task. Possibly this

115

additional burden was too much to expect of Freud. He
was, after all, having it difficult enough putting
forward the image of humanity encompassed by psychoanalysis. Why borrow more trouble? But I do not
think he avoided attacking the philosophy of science
eagerly embraced by Brüke, Breuer, and Fliess out of
concern for adding weight to his overburdened load. I
think Freud was just not much drawn to abstract
analyses of concepts in an impersonal sense. He
always finds latent contents taking him far beyond the
bounds of rationality, into the personal and the defensive uses of mentation. In the Freud-Jung letters
(see McGuire, 1974) we find the debate over the nature
of libido (and other issues) slipping again and again
into the supposed underlying personal reasons for why
one man or the other is holding to a position (see esp.
pp. 297-300). The ad hominem runs amuck in analytical
therapeutics. This does not mean that ad hominem
arguments are inappropriate in psychoanalysis. Doubt-
less we do behave in this manner--finding masking
reasons for contending what we really want to say or
do for quite other reasons. Granting this truism, is
it not also possible that "disinterested" philosophical
analyses of assumptions like "What is the nature of
libido?" or "Do we really need a libido construct?" are
meaningful in their own right--or, if one prefers, at
their own "level" of awareness?

Surely the answer here is obvious. If Freud had
been more prepared to examine philosophical assumptions
of the natural science of his day, he might and I believe he would have fashioned a more viable theory of
personality than we have at present in the name of
psychoanalysis. His theory of illness would not have
fallen into the quagmire of supposed "fixations of
libido" at earlier life periods, to which the personality organization regresses in hope of recouping
this precious (non-) "stuff." He might have remained
with his initial theoretical inclinations, of describing people as caught up in their dialectically conflicting intentions (wishes), as affirming one course
of life or another, usually with second thoughts, and
often with regrets over the compromised course actually
taken. His antithetical ideas and counter-will notions
seem to me far more appropriate as descriptions of
human behavior than the pseudo-reductive formulation
he arrived at.

In closing, I would like to state that philosophy has immense implications for personality theory and psychotherapy, as it has for all aspects of human experience. I would go further and suggest that philosophy could indeed be expected to bring its wisdom to the actual practice of psychotherapy. Of course, I believe that any philosophical examination in psychotherapy must take the affective and the emotional into consideration. We must not fool ourselves into believing that we are only "rationl" animals--the reverse of Freud's predilections. I have always thought that Jung had the right idea in placing rationality on the side of feelings as well as rational thoughts. Feelings are just as evaluative and/or judgmental as are thoughts. All of which brings us back to the fact that it demands a final-cause phrasing to capture true evaluations, true judgments "for the sake of" some standard, reason, affective preference, and so on. Teleology is central to a proper conceptualization of human nature, a fact which should not surprise philosophers since it is they who--centuries past--first made us aware of this fact.

It is unfortunate that Freud never seems to have appreciated the philosophically dated arguments that Brucke, Breuer, and Fliess were advancing. I think that today, looking back, we can marvel at the deftness of his solution to the problem facing him even as we appreciate that in modern approaches to the philosophy of science these maneuvers are no longer called for. In the future we can retain the Freudian insights regarding the telic nature of mind even as we <u>drop</u> the outmoded reliance on constancy-principle reductionism.

THE ROLE OF PHILOSOPHY IN FIVE KINDS OF PSYCHOTHERAPEUTIC SYSTEMS

Edith Weisskopf-Joelson

There are many ways in which we can interpret the world which surrounds us. The great variety of interpretive systems created by humans has been given many names; they have been called philosophies, world views, Weltanschauungen, phenomenological fields (Lewin, 1935; Snygg & Combs, 1949), belief systems, perceptual houses (Hobbs, 1962). Among these terms my favorite is "perceptual houses" which I shall use throughout this chapter.

All philosophies are perceptual houses, but not all perceptual houses are philosophies. Some perceptual houses are rarely called philosophies because they address themselves to a narrow topic rather than to a broad area. The belief in the desirability of prohibition is an example of such a perceptual house or perhaps a perceptual "cabin."

The effect on our lives of the perceptual houses in which we live cannot be overestimated (Weisskopf-Joelson, 1953, 1968). It almost seems that "what is" is less important than our perception of it. As Epictetus wrote, "Men are disturbed not by things, but by the view they take of them" (1955, p. 19). Consider the following examples:

A young woman who had the desire and ability to become a United States Senator might have perceived herself as neurotic and inferior in the fifties, but as healthy and superior in the late sixties. The women's liberation movement, a perceptual house, has altered the self-concept of many women in the deepest possible sense.
    . . .
A Chinese comic strip tells about a young girl, Dai Bee-lun, who saved the lives of three small children by pushing them off the tracks a split second before a runaway freight car was about to hit them. At this crucial moment, she remembered the teaching of Chairman Mao-Tse-tung: "When we die for the people, it is a worthy death." The children remained unharmed, but Dai Bee-lun lost one arm. She said: "Don't feel sorry for me. I still have one arm to write the thoughts of Chairman Mao. I can still serve the

people." Both doctors and nurses praised her highly. (New York Times Magazine, February 20, 1972, 12-15). Thus, a political perceptual house turned despair into happiness.

. . .

Sister Theresa, a missionary nun, dying from tuberculosis around Easter time, said: "This is a good time to be on the cross!" A religious perceptual house transformed a tragedy into a triumph.

. . .

For the purpose of discussing the function of perceptual houses in psychotherapy, I shall define five types of psychotherapy which differ with regard to the role played, in their theories and practices, by perceptual houses.

A. Psychodynamic Therapies are therapies in which the psyche is seen as divided into various parts, for example, the conscious and the unconscious, where therapy consists in correcting the imbalance between the parts in a disturbed individual. The term "psychodynamic" suggest that psychic energies are moving and changing places during therapy as an effect of interpretations by the therapist of the patient's verbal and nonverbal behavior.

Freudian psychoanalysis (1933) is the best known example of a Psychodynamic Therapy. It is, in part, based on the theory that the etiology of neurosis is incomplete repression, during childhood, of guilt producing or otherwise threatening events. Since the repression is incomplete, the patient may suffer from a variety of negative emotions which seem to defy explanation because they are responses to repressed material unknown to both patient and therapist. Thus, it becomes the task of the therapist to help the patient regain consciousness of the repressed threat. As a result, the neurotic emotions become visibly connected to threatening memories. While the threat could not be tolerated by the small child, it can be tolerated by the mature adult. For example, an adult may suffer from free-floating, unexplainable guilt feelings. Analysis may reveal that the patient, as a boy, hated his father. The father subsequently died

120

in an accident. The boy, engaging in magical thinking common among young children, thought his hatred had killed his father. Only after the guilt producing stimuli have become conscious, can the patient evaluate them in terms of adult thought processes. Now he knows that thoughts do not kill and this awareness will remove his neurotic feelings of guilt although some healthy guilt feelings about hating his father may remain.

The reader should keep in mind that the above is only one of many possible examples of psychodynamic theories and even this example is highly oversimplified.

The question which concerns us here is whether a perceptual house, a philosophical system, plays a role in the psychotherapeutic effect of Psychodynamic Therapies. Psychoanalysis, is, of course, a perceptual house or a psychological philosophy. But it is a perceptual house which the therapist must study, adopt, and apply to the patient. The patient will not be cured by becoming a true believer in psychoanalytic theory. He may be cured by having this theory applied to him. However, when I speak, in this chapter, about the therapeutic effect of philosophies, or perceptual houses, I focus on the therapeutic effect of the patient, adopting a perceptual house, whereby specific features of this perceptual house become healing agents for the patient. Thus, we may say that psychodynamic therapies do not heal through the adoption of perceptual houses.

However, all psychotherapies, including psychodynamic ones, may heal by way of perceptual houses, in a more general sense, insofar as many patients adopt the basic philosophy underlying the therapy they receive. As a consequence, their world is perceived as structured, interpreted, explained and consistent, and the mere fact of living in a phenomenologically ordered world may bring about some therapeutic effects as a by-product.

B. Didactic Therapies. These therapies consist in teaching and helping the patient adopt a specific perceptual house. While in Psychodynamic Therapies the therapeutic effect of adopting a perceptual house is viewed as a by-product, in Didactic Therapies

this adoption is viewed as the main source of therapy.
However, the perceptual house is not a deeply felt,
passionate, coherent view of human existence. Instead, it is a series of relatively unrelated, cognitive, pragmatic hypotheses.

Rational-Emotive Therapy (Ellis, 1973) may serve
as an example of a Didactic Therapy.

Rationale-Emotive Therapy is based on the belief
that there are no legitimate reasons for feeling highly anxious, guilty or worried. Negative emotions of
this kind are based on irrational ideas, on unverifiable hypotheses which can be replaced by rational
ideas through educational procedures.

Below are some examples of these irrational ideas,
each followed by the rational idea with which the
patient is taught to replace his faulty thoughts
(Mahoney, 1974).

1. The idea that it is a dire necessity for an
adult to be loved by everyone for everything he
does - instead of concentrating on his own self-
respect, on winning approval for practical purposes, and on loving rather than being loved.
(p. 171)

2. The idea that certain acts are awful or
wicked, and that people who perform such acts
should be severely punished - instead of the
idea that certain acts are inappropriate or anti-
social, and that people who perform such acts are
behaving stupidly, ignorantly, or neurotically
and would be better helped to change. (p. 171)

3. The idea that it would be horrible when things
are not the way one would like them to be -
instead of the idea that it is too bad, that one
would better try to change or control conditions
so that they become more satisfactory, and, if
that is not possible, one had better temporarily
accept their existence. (p. 171)

The actual psychotherapy is carried out in diadic
or group interactions in which patients are taught that
the false hypotheses which they hold are irrational.
They are also taught, through verbal interaction and

122

homework assignments, to accept the rational corrections of their irrational thoughts. The homework consists in engaging in activities which are disturbing to the patients because, according to rational-emotive theory, they approach these activities in terms of irrational hypotheses. They might be asked to look for a job, to date, to return to a spouse whom they left. But, when engaging in these activities, they are now assigned to approach them with their recently learned rational hypotheses in mind.

Some of my criticisms of this school is the basic foundation which implies that knowing the good is doing the good, an assumption which is contradicted by introspection, the clinical experience of depth psychologists, the observation of obsessive-compulsive people, and the psychological wisdom of great writers (Goethe, Shakespeare, Dostoevsky). In addition, the meaning of "irrational" is almost exclusively defined by the concommitance of irrational ideas and emotional disturbances. Thus, the "discovery" that irrational ideas cause emotional disturbances appears to be a tautology.

Furthermore, on a more subjective level, the presupposition that anxiety and guilt are always "irrational" emotions is opposed to my own philosophy which holds that Angst and guilt, are, in many cases, necessary, helpful and deeply spiritual emotions.

Rational-Emotive Therapy seems like a good example of a Didactic Psychotherapy. "Didactic" can be defined as "intended to convey instruction and information" and this is what Rational-Emotive Therapy does. Moreover, it focuses on the intellectual aspect of disturbed people, on their hypotheses, on their irrationalities, on their thoughts. However, other writers seem to disagree with me on the merely cognitive nature of Rational-Emotive Therapy; they feel it produces deep philosophical change and strives for thorough emotional reorientation (Mahoney, 1974). If this is the case, then Rational-Emotive Therapy would have to be subsumed under the next heading of Conversional Therapies.

In conclusion, the rational ideas which the client is taught can be viewed as philosophies or perceptual houses. Thus, in didactic therapies, philosophies are viewed as the main therapeutic factors.

C. <u>Conversional</u> "<u>Therapies</u>." Even more than
other kinds of therapies, Conversional "Therapies"
are sought not only by people with neurotic symptoms
but also by "healthy" people who want to grow, to
find a purpose in life, to be creative, to improve
their relationships to others. They differ from
Didactic Therapies insofar as they do not speak of
rational hypotheses, but of health-engendering beliefs
and faiths which the client is hoped to adopt. While
Didactic Therapies are based on the presupposition "I
think, therefore I feel," Conversional "Therapies"
presupposition is closer to "I believe, therefore I
feel."

In Conversional "Therapy," the side effect of
Psychodynamic Theories, namely the acquisition of a
perceptual house, becomes the main purpose of "therapy"
in quotes because, as some of my illustrations will
show, conversional perceptual houses are often called
"philosophies" rather than "therapies." However,
one could be a "patient" of Albert Camus, of Jean
Paul Sartre, of Friedrich Nietzsche, or Soren
Kierkegaard, of Rollo May, of Martin Heidegger. Thus
in this sense, the concepts "therapy" and "philosophy"
are often interchangeable.

Most of the above thinkers can be subsumed under
the heading of existential philosophers. Existential
philosophy lends itself as a basis of "therapy" for
the sick and for the well, and as an example of
Conversional "Therapies." Since existential philosophies differ from philosopher to philosopher, I shall
use, as illustrations, the thoughts of individual
philosophers rather than existential thought in general.

First, I shall describe some parts of the perceptual house of the existential philosopher, novelist
and playwright Albert Camus. Camus changed his views
in the course of his life; thus, what I am describing
is a temporary philosophy held by Camus. It suggests
that a very negative, seemingly pessimistic philosophy
can be therapeutic.

Camus (1955) speaks of the human condition as
"the absurd" and of the ideal person as "the absurd
man."

Descriptions of the aspects of our existence

which are absurd are scattered through Camus'
writings. I have gathered them together and shall
present them systematically in what follows. The
absurd is brought about by the following aspects of
the human condition.

1. Death is our worst enemy. If life inescap-
ably ends in death, everything loses its importance--
nothing matters. How can we hope, long for, or con-
template the future joyfully if we know that, as our
hopes are fulfilled, time advances and carries us
closer, and closer, towards death?

2. The world does not provide us with a meaning
of our lives. "Rising, streetcar, four hours in the
office or the factory, meal, streetcar, four hours of
work, meal, sleep, and Monday, Tuesday, Wednesday,
Thursday, Friday and Saturday according to the same
rhythm...But one day the 'why' arises..." An answer
to the "why" is never forthcoming.

3. The non-human world is alien to us, it does
not have feelings and thoughts as we do; it is
characterized by an "implacable otherness." If the
universe could love and suffer as we do, there would
be unity. Or, there would be unity if we "were a
tree among trees, a cat among animals..." but we are
irreversibly severed from the world we live in.

4. The human world, too, is alien to us. We
can never truly apprehend the thoughts and feelings of
others.

5. We are severed and estranged from ourselves.
We look in the mirror and meet a stranger.

6. We are filled with nostalgia to understand
the universe in which we live. But we can do so
only to a very limited extent.

7. We yearn for a single principle to explain
the universe, but we find that no such principle
exists.

Thus, the mind desires and the world disappoints.
What can be done about all these deplorable aspects of
the human condition? In answering this question Camus
depicts an attitude toward the absurd which he considers desirable on a priori basis, and he describes

and advocates this attitude with extreme passion; it
is the attitude held by "the absurd man."

The rules which govern the life of the absurd
man can be summarized in three words: "Do not cheat."
Live solely with what you know. Preserve your honesty.
Do not embrace illusions which go beyond the knowable,
such as religious illusions. Religions ask man to
make a leap toward faith, but Camus says "Do not leap"
for leaping is a way of cheating, a subterfuge which
destroys integrity. The absurd man remains on the
"dizzying crest before the leap." The absurd "must
not be forgotten. It must be clung to because the
whole consequence of life can depend on it." Do not
leave the desert behind. "Preserve the very thing
that crushes you. This implies a total absence of
hope....Everything that destroys, conjures away, or
exorcises these requirements---ruins the absurd."
The absurd man decides to lead "a life without consolation." He does not elude the absurd by "trickery
of those who live not for life itself but for some
great idea that will transcend it, refine it, give it
a meaning, and betray it. (Italics mine). He does
not try to be cured but, instead, to live with his
ailment."

The central question of Camus' essay "Does the
absurd condition of man justify suicide?" can now be
answered. The absurd man will not commit suicide
because he is intent on preserving the absurd, and
suicide would resolve absurdity and make it vanish.
"It is essential to die unreconciled and not of one's
own free will."

Is the philosophy of the absurd a philosophy
of renunciation, of passively accepting one's lot
without fight? Camus' answer is "No." The absurd man
is characterized by passionate revolt against fate, by
continual struggle and defiance without the slightest
hope of victory. "The absurd has meaning only insofar
as it is not agreed to."

So much about the absurd. Incidentally, one way
in which the difference between the didactic Rational-
Emotive Therapy and the Conversional "Therapy" of
Camus can be illuminated is by the difference in style:
Didactic systems teach, and teaching is traditionally
done in clear, logical, non-dramatic, non-passionate

and non-metaphorical language. In contrast, existential systems convert, and conversion is traditionally done in dramatic, passionate and often metaphorical language. Camus' language sounds like a child of many parents: of a philosopher, a novelist, a poet, a preacher and a <u>psychotherapist</u>.

The latter brings us to the question which we now have to ask ourselves: How can a philosophy of the absurd be psychotherapeutic? Or, more generally speaking, can a negative view of life be health-engendering? A negative view of life might help us see our personal problems as an aspect of the human condition; it might help us see the problems of other people as similar to our own and, thus, mitigate our loneliness. Since no one can entirely escape the anxieties of life, giving them an official status in a shared world view changes the anxious view of life from a private one to a shared one.

Moreover, the absurd viewpoint is grim, but by acceptance of the grim aspects of life we might avoid disappointments caused by unwarranted hopes. The absurd man will not be sad about being sad because he knows that sadness is an inexorable aspect of life.

It is especially important to become aware of the inexorable, anxiety provoking, and, therefore, repressed of existence. This awareness produces "existential anxiety" i.e., anxiety about the <u>real</u> dangers and tragedies of life. The repression of existential anxiety creates neurotic or unrealistic anxiety. Existentially anxious people are allegedly at a great advantage compared with neurotically anxious ones, because constant awareness of the human condition enables them to shape their lives realistically within the limitations imposed by this condition.

Now I wish to discuss some aspects of another philosophy which is more often viewed as a school of therapy, namely Logotherapy, a school originated by Frankl (1969). It represents a typical example of the kind of therapy which I have called conversional. It is especially interesting to compare Logotherapy with Camus' philosophy of the absurd, because the two schools are in many ways on opposite ends of a continuum.

127

The absurd man is defiant, proud and unwilling to accept any consolation. What keeps him alive is--as it were--the attempt to show the universe that he does not need the gifts which it refuses to give. Without any ties of values, to ideals, to people, or to nature, he is free and can enjoy the pleasures of the moment in a grim fashion.

Well, some people can live that way and if they are artists, they will create grim and heroic paintings, poems, stories, or music.

But not all people are able to live an absurd existence. For many of us the absurd leads to unbearable despair, especially since it cannot and must not be filled with meaning, because any meaning is viewed an illusion. Despair about meaninglessness (existential anxiety) is the very condition which Logotherapy attempts to alleviate.

Logotherapy does not alleviate existential anxiety by changing the world, the society, the family, but by changing our perception of all the above. In other words, Logotherapy builds a new perceptual house which has the power to counteract the absurd.

When the dull routine of rising, working, eating, sleeping, raises, one day, the question "Why?", then the Logotherapist will answer the question maybe by using Nietzsche's words:

"Whoever has a reason for living can endure almost any mode of life." (Cf. Frankl, 1969, p. 121)

If we have a purpose, a goal in life, then dull routines will not seem so dull because they are known to be a part of one or more overriding purposes or goals to which we have dedicated our lives.

Frankl calls these purposes "meaning." We cannot arbitrarily ascribe meaning to our lives since meaning already exists, in some mysterious way, and must be discovered by our own intuition. To discover the meaning of our lives is, according to Frankl, our strongest yearning; it is stronger than the yearning for pleasure or power.

The meaning of every person's life is unique,

i.e., it differs from one person to the other.   In Buber's (1958) words

> Every person born into the world represents some-
> thing new, something that never existed before,
> something original and unique.   It is the duty of
> every person to know that there has never been
> anyone like him in the world.   Every single man
> is a new thing in the world and is called upon to
> fulfill his particularity in this world.   (pp.
> 139-140)

Again: now rising, working, eating, sleeping
does not seem so absurd anymore!   It might be done to
support one's childrne, to send them to college and
this might be a big part of the riser's, worker's
eater's, and sleeper's meaning of life.   Or, the
meaning might be writing a book and, as Frankl and
Buber say, there is no one in the world who can write
a book exactly like that one person who has to rise,
work, eat, and sleep from Monday to Friday, or even
to Sunday in order to do it.   So what?   Absurdity
capitulates when meaning appears on the scene.

Camus might have called Frankl's concept of meaning a consoling illusion or philosophical suicide.
But is not the philosophy of the absurd as well as
Logotherapy a subjective perceptual house?   The
existence of Frankl's meaning cannot be empirically
verified or falsified; instead it rests on subjective
intuition and feelings.   But so does the absurd.   Is it
true that death makes every thing lose its importance?
Many philosophers believe the opposite to be true.   Is
it true that nature negates us?   (Incidentally: what
does it mean?)   Would we be better off if we "were
a tree among trees, a cat among animal...?"   De-
gustibus non est discutandum (One man's meat is another
man's poison).   Can we never apprehend the thoughts
and feelings of others?   Do we meet a stranger when we
look in the mirror?

Obviously, Camus' and Frankl's perceptual houses
are, as all perceptual houses (by definition), two
different ways of looking at reality both of which
are compatible with reality but transcend reality.   The
terms "true" or "false" cannot be applied to them, but
the terms "therapeutic" or "not therapeutic" can.   I
hypothesized that both philosophies could be therapeutic even though they contradict each other with

regard to their content. Perhaps, different philosophies are therapeutic for different kinds of
people. If so, the relationship between personality,
sex, social class, age, etc. and optimal perceptual
house may yield interesting and applicable results.

In concluding this section, I would like to repeat that Conversional "Therapies" aim at converting
the client to a therapeutic perceptual house, whereby
the therapeutic effect of such a conversion is viewed
as the main effect rather than merely a byproduct.

Moreover, I wish to suggest a yet unmentioned
common characteristic of the last two types of therapy,
namely of Didactic and Conversional Therapies. In
both cases, the basic texts of these therapies can
serve several purposes at the same time. These books
contain the "messages" which make up the perceptual
houses. Thus, the therapist can use them to be taught
or to be converted, and simultaneously to learn how
to teach or convert the client. Both therapist and
client have to learn the same message. Should a
therapist be unavailable, the client could possibly
cure himself by reading the text. In contrast, this
is not the case with regard to psychodynamic therapies.
The patient cannot be cured by reading books on
"How to practice psychoanalysis." These are books
which have only one purpose, namely to tell the
analyst what to do to or with the patient when psy-
choanalysing him. Thus, the textbooks of Didactic
and Conversional Therapies resemble bibles, while
those of psychoanalysis resemble those sections in a
textbook on surgery which teach how to do surgery on
a part of the body which cannot be seen or reached by
the patient.

D. Ecological Therapies. Ecological Therapies
are based on the assumption that the client's complaints are consequences of an unfavorable environment, and that it is the environment which needs to
be changed in addition to, or rather than the individual. One example of Ecological Therapy is Radical Therapy which is based on the political philosophy of Karl Marx (Brown, 1973).

It is a basic tenet of Radical Therapy that individual therapy is frequently an undesirable procedure because it maintains the status quo by

adjusting clients to an oppressive society. In order
to cure the contemporary epidemic of alienation,
boredom, depression, meaninglessness, it is necessary
to change society as a whole. Therefore, Radical
Therapists tend to be political activists by engaging
in shared opposition of a non-militant or even of a
militant nature against the establishment and by in-
ducing their clients to do the same.

These tenets may seem somewhat inappropriate to
most readers for many reasons, one being that books
like the present one are mostly read by somewhat
privileged people who do not find our society so unacceptable that it would need to be changed in toto.
Therefore, it might make it easier to evoke some empathy with Radical Therapy if we focused upon a
society other than our own, a society about which
most of us would agree that it might be the cause of
most evil experienced by its members.

Nazi Germany might be such a society: Let us
imagine an anti-Nazi therapist practicing in Germany
during the Nazi regime. A client in his early
twenties comes to see him with complaints of a general
nature: unhappiness, insomnia, inefficiency on the
job, free-floating feelings of guilt. The therapist's
first thought (which he would, in most cases, not
immediately communicate to the client) would be:

"Is this not a perfectly normal response to the
unbearable society in which you and I live?"

Moreover, if the client is strong, healthy, experienced in leadership and political work, a further
thought might occur to the therapist:

"Why does this young man not join the underground
movement?" (a thought which he would not communicate
to the client since such a dangerous decision cannot
be made by anybody other than the client.)

Radical therapists see the societies of the western world as equally oppressive as the Nazi society.
This oppression is viewed as the basic cause of
emotional disturbance. Oppression can be defined as a
coercion of human beings by covert or overt force.

However, in order to become a power that causes
neurotic disturbance, oppression must be accompanied

by mystification. Mystification is the deception of oppressed people regarding the fact that they are oppressed and regarding the manner in which this oppression is exerted. The mystification may be created consciously or unconsciously by a group of people, called the oppressors, or by the mores of the society at large.

I shall describe the basic techniques used by Radical Therapists to help oppressed people, using women as an example of an oppressed group. In the fifties, before the new women's liberation movement started, most white, middle class young women made it their lives' goal to get married and raise a family. The men whom they dated, the parents who oversaw their dating, the media (including TV commercials) and last, not least, most psychotherapists spread the message that being a wife and mother was the only fulfillment of a woman's life. But, soon other voices became audible in the form of feminist publications, saying that the bliss of the feminine role was a myth rather than a fact. As these voices became increasingly loud, a strange thing happened: Many women who were previously convinced that they had found bliss and fulfillment in the homemakers' roles began to "realize" that their bliss was an illusion, that the glamour of marriage and motherhood was an oppressive slogan used by man to keep women in their place.

Doubtful and dissatisfied women met in groups, often under the leadership of feminist therapists (always women) many of whom are a special subgroup of Radical Therapists.

Many of these feminist therapists' dealing with disturbed women are guided by the following formulas (Agel, 1971):

Oppression + Mystification = Emotional Disrubrance
Oppression + Awareness = Anger
Anger + Contact = Liberation

The same formulas are used by many other Radical Therapists.

The formulas say that if a person is oppressed, without knowing that, or how, she is oppressed, she may become emotionally disturbed. If by the guidance of a feminist therapist she becomes aware of her

132

oppression and its nature, her emotional disturbance
will change into realistic anger. Then she is en-
couraged to seek contact with other angry women, and
thus, to become a member of a revolutionary group.
Now she and her peers have found a manner in which
they can fight for their own mental health and,
simultaneously, for the mental health of their society.

The above suggests a connection between the
Marxist foundation of Radical Psychology and the new
women's liberation movement, even though large portions
of the new women's liberation movement do not view
themselves as related to Marxism.

Next I wish to give at least some idea what a
Radical Therapist does in addition to leading feminist
therapy groups.

First, a dramatic and probably atypical example
(Agel, pp. 199-209). In 1970, a group of physicians
and other health workers from the Medical Liberation
Front and about 50 black and white members of the
community seized all the offices and 120 (out of 800)
beds of St. Luke's Hospital, located one block away
from the Harlem Ghetto, in order to set up walk-in
heroin and detoxification units. This was done as a
response to what was viewed, by the militant group,
as unethical practices of the hospital administration:
In spite of St. Luke's being a publicly founded institution, its priorities were not the needs of the
community. Instead, the priorities were research and
teaching; thus, the hospital was seen as publicly
funded but privately serving. The hospital administration did not call the police for protection against
the invaders presumably because it wanted to avoid an
investigation. The event was given wide press and
television coverage and thus the hospital was increasingly pressured to meet the demands for addiction
services.

Mental health workers speak and write much about
the fast growing multitude of their techniques, but
the militant takeover of facilities is usually not
mentioned among them.

Brown (1973) gives a brief summary of other radical activities: "Radical therapy is any of the following: organizing a community to seize control of the

way it's run; helping a brother or sister through a crisis; rooting out our own chauvinism and mercilessly exposing it in others; focusing on the social dimensions of oppression and not on intrapsychic depression, fear, anger, and so on; organizing against the war, against polluting industries, against racist practice; developing a political/therapy center for young people; teaching students psychology like it is; refusing to be manipulated and co-opted by (those) who heap praise on your head" (p. 519) in order to seize control over you.

In conclusion, Radical Therapy, as an example of Ecological Therapies, uses a political philosophy for therapeutic purposes in several ways. The therapist, who is a believer in the philosophy, converts the clients to the philosophy and encourages them to engage in the actions prescribed by the philosophy. This is therapeutic, first, because it creates a perceptual house for the client as all therapies do (overtly or covertly), second, because it gives meaning to the clients' lives and thus spurs them to action, third, because it makes them members of congenial communities and fourth, because the action suggested by the philosophy is said to remove, or help remove, the cause of the clients' psychic pains.

E. Catalytic Therapies. A therapeutic school can be called a catalytic if the therapist functions as a catalyst rather than as an active agent. The word "catalyst" is taken from the field of chemistry. A chemical is called a catalyst if it brings about or facilitates a chemical reaction without participating in the reaction. Similarly, the catalytic therapist offers the client neither interpretations, nor advice, or conversion to a perceptual house. Instead, clients work out their own problems and the therapist facilitates their work by comments showing genuine respect and understanding.

Rogers (1951) Client-Centered Therapy exemplifies Catalytic Therapy. Rogers believes that human beings have a natural tendency to grow and to actualize their potentialities, and that they will do so if they are "planted into the right soil." The catalytic therapist is like a gardner who provides the soil and the water and lets the apple seed grow into an apple tree rather than trying to change it into a peach tree.

134

The question which concerns us in this chapter
is: does the catalytic therapist use a philosophical
system when engaging in this kind of therapy? The
official answer is "no." Rogers' procedure is, of
course, based on an extensive philosophy but he does
not present this philosophy to his clients, and does
not suggest that they make it their own. Instead,
he creates an atmosmphere in which clients can develop
their own philosophy.

But, alas, is it possible to interact with other
human beings without exerting some influence on them?
The following example shows how easily thoughts are
transferred between persons who are close to each
other.

A Rogerian therapist reports the following conver-
sation with a young woman. The client speaks first:

"In seeking an alternative to teaching
I have thought of a more practical occupation
than gardening. With my savings I'd take a six
months' course in domestic science. Then I would
try to get employment as a housekeeper. Next to
gardening I would like best to look after a
house."

"Whose house?"

"Oh, perhaps some married couple who were
out all the time and left everything up to me."

She becomes silent for several minutes. I
do not speak. Finally she continues:

"I suppose you are thinking that it ought to
be my house. That I ought to get married."

The therapist, be it noted, made no critical
comment; the patient simply interpreted his
silence as criticism. Had the therapist given
voice merely to an "m-hm," she would have continued with her fancying. (De Gracia, 1952,
p. 85)

Thus, philosophies are hard to contain. A
slight movement of the therapist's brow, a nearly
invisible smile can induce clients at crossroads to

135

choose a path which may save them or one which may destroy them.

CONCLUSION

With the above considerations in mind one can only marvel at the creative power of the human spirit.

With some overdramatization one could say that human beings have achieved considerable independence from their destiny because they can build perceptual houses, which can change isolation into intimacy, meaninglessness into meaning, self-hatred into self-satisfaction, tragedy into triumph, and as my last chapter will show, death into eternal life.

RELIGION AND PSYCHOTHERAPY

RELIGION AND PSYCHOTHERAPY

The issue of the relation between psychotherapy and religion has already been mentioned in several of the preceeding essays, having its origins in the very birth of modern psychotherapy. The role of the psychotherapist as a kind of secular pastoral counselor places him and his profession in the position of sometimes reinforcing and sometimes competing with traditional religious values and guidance. Both religion and psychotherapy claim to be concerned with the health of the psyche' but from very different metaphysical perspectives. Most psychotherapeutic models are based upon a naturalistic metaphysic while most religions are supernatural in orientation.

In their more extreme forms psychotherapy and religion have condemned one another for false and illusory practices and beliefs, each accusing the other of compounding pathologies and obscuring rather than facilitating recognition of "the truth that sets us free." Religions and psychotherapies, however, come in many different kinds and the debate between them is only a reflection of the debate that goes on within each between competing ideologies. Among the various beliefs and practices of psychotherapies and religions there are those which are no doubt more conducive to the development of healthy psyche's and those which are not. The question is, how are the healthy to be distinguished from the unhealthy and how is the relation between even "healthy" religions and psychotherapies to be understood?

At least this much seems to be clear for the present. Neither psychotherapy nor religion can, prima facie, rule the other out of court. Neither is justified in arbitrarily ignoring or dismissing the apparent success and influence of the other any more than they should overlook each other's and their own faults and failures. Insofar as psychotherapy tends to focus exclusively on the psyche's state of health in the here-and-now it can make no claims, positive or negative, concerning its survival or "health" in the here-after, nor can it predicate itself on an assumed solution to this ancient question. Religion on the other hand, should be sensitive to and respectful of the insights and methods of psychotherapy, for whether or not the psyche' survives the here-and-now, there is no reason to believe that an unhealthy psyche' in the here-and-now will automatically be healthy in the here-after. Whether we survive in the here-after or only in the here-and-now we are still possessed of but one psyche' and until the verdict is conclusively in, the dictates of a coherent and wholistic approach to the health of our psyche's demands the recognition, if not cooperation, of psychotherapy and religion each of the other.

Just as it would be misleading and potentially dangerous to confuse the kind of foundations involved in science, philosophy and psychotherapy so too would it be misleading and dangerous for religion and psychotherapy to attempt to play the role of the other. As the first essay of this section argues, psychotherapy cannot be identified solely with medicine, but neither can it be so identified with religion. It can claim for itself the authority of neither but must stand on its own as an art related to but distinct from both. Psychotherapy's identity crisis is, like any identity crisis, one which cannot be solved by attempting to take on the identity of another but only by acknowledging its true origins and accepting the responsibility of developing an identity of its own.

As argued in our first essay of this section, there is in particular a danger of psychotherapy playing the role of religion but masquerading as medicine. The danger lies in the social and political sanctioning of a particular philosophical world view in the name of "health." Such claims could and have threatened to outlaw ideologies and life styles at variance with its own value presuppositions in the name of promoting "mental health." Here it is crucial that the essentially philosophical foundations of all psychotherapeutic models be acknowledged and made clearly manifest.

The recognition of the essentially naturalistic or philosophically rationalistic character of the foundations of psychotherapy raises an important question about its relation to the essentially supernaturalistic faith supported foundations of religion. How is dialogue and mutual recognition, let alone cooperation, even possible between two such apparently diametrically opposed metaphysical world views?

140

The answer to this question is not as difficult as it may at first seem. Its solution lies in the proper understanding of the relation between philosophy and religion. For, while philosophy must continue always to seek natural explanations for the problems and questions with which she is confronted, even she rests upon a kind of faith that such explanations are possible. Philosophy cannot make dogmatic pronouncements concerning as yet unanswered questions and remain philosophical. The relation between philosophy and religion might be described as the clash between faith in the possibility of knowledge and faith in the unknown. But, it must always be remembered that it is faith in the possibility of knowledge and not the claim of knowledge itself which constitutes the foundation of philosophy.

In other words, psychotherapy, if it is to remain true to its philosophical origins, must remain silent or at least objective about as yet unanswered issues of faith though like philosophy, it should be resolute in its persistence to find a rational explanation. This means that psychotherapy must investigate and take seriously, though it need not agree with, the claims made on behalf of religious faith, for that faith is itself something which requires explanation. The greatest philosophical sin--the sin against wisdom would be to represent as solved or as known that which is really as yet unknown. To do so would indeed be to confuse philosophy with religion and to repudiate precisely that which distinguishes psychotherapy from religious practice and ideology.

Though presented from somewhat different perspectives, the second and third essays of this section represent legitimate philosophical approaches to clarifying the relation between religion and psychotherapy.

The first of the pair investigates basic values in humanistic psychotherapy and major elements of the Judeo-Christian biblical tradition with a view toward mediating some of the differences and misunderstandings concerning the relation between the two. Its focus is on helping clinicians to understand, though not necessarily agree with, the religious perspectives of their clients as a kind of minimal reconciliation of religion and psychotherapy.

141

The second essay of the pair provides us with a close philosophical analysis of the concept of the "self" in humanistic psychotherapies and in the Judeo-Christian religious tradition, warning that a complete reconciliation is not possible without major concessions on the part of one or the other. Here the focus is upon pastoral counselors who may have adopted techniques of humnaistic therapies without realizing the consequences for potential conflict with traditional religious doctrines.

The last essay of the section, and of the collection, turns the question around completely to investigate the therapeutic aspects of religions and or political philosophies--how can and do religious and political philosophies lead to meaning, happiness and fulfillment? The author invites her readers to attempt to experience through empathy what <u>faith</u> feels like and its power in "healing" those for whom it provides a sense of place and belonging.

These essays are not included here with the intention of collapsing religion into psychotherapy or <u>vice versa</u> but only as examples of the kind of study and dialogue that must be begun if either is to find its proper relation to the other in realizing its own identity.

PSYCHOTHERAPY: MEDICINE, RELIGION, AND POWER

Thomas S. Szasz

The controversy over whether psychotherapy belongs to medicine or religion is not new. Freud and
Jung devoted a great deal of attention to this problem,
claiming psychotherapy sometimes for medicine, sometimes for religion. Their ambivalence about this
question reflects, in part, their uncertainty about
the nature of the mental disorders they were "treating",
and in part their unwillingness, because of its practical implications, to commit themselves exclusively to
either a medical or a moral perspective on psychotherapy.

Freud was equally eloquent in arguing that mental
diseases were organic disorders whose proper treatment was chemical, and in arguing that they were psychological problems whose proper treatment was pastoral.
For example, in 1914, Freud asserts: "All our pro-
visional ideas in psychology will presumably some day
be based on an organic substructure. This makes it
probable that it is special substances and chemical processes which perform the operations of. . .special
pscyhical forces." (Freud, 1914, p. 78) In 1930, he
declares: "The hope of the future lies in organic
chemistry or access to it through endocrinology. This
future is still far distant, but one should study
analytically every case of psychosis because this knowledge will one day guide the chemical therapy." (Freud,
1930, p. 449) And in 1938, in An Outline of Psycho-
Analysis, he reiterates this view and extends it to
encompass all mental diseases: "The future may teach
us to exercise a direct influence, by means of particular chemical substances, on the amounts of energy and
their distribution in the neural apparatus. It may be
that there are other still undreamt-of possibilities
of therapy. But for the moment we have nothing better
at our disposal than the technique of psychoanalysis."
(Frued, 1938, p. 182) These excerpts show us Freud as
the cryptobiologist and the secret believer in the
chemical treatment of mental diseases.

There was, however, another side to Freud, a side
that looked upon psychoanalysis not as a poor substitute
for a future chemical miracle cure, but as a valuable
discovery for probing the unconscious and as an in-
valuable therapy for the neuroses. For example, in
1919, Freud writes that the analyst's task is

143

"to bring to the patient's knowledge the unconscious, repressed impulses existing in him". (Freud, 1919, p. 159) In 1928, he repeats his "wish to protect analysis from the doctors (and the priests)." (Freud/ Pfister, p. 126) And in 1927, in his essay on lay (nonmedical) analysis, he declares, "I have assumed that psychoanalysis is not a specialized branch of medicine. I cannot see how it is possible to dispute this." (Freud, 1927, p. 252) But if psychoanalysis is not a branch of medicine, what is it a branch of? This is Freud's answer: "The words, 'secular pastoral worker,' might well serve as a general formula for describing the function of the analyst. . . We do not seek to bring (the patient) relief by receiving him into the catholic, protestant, or socialist community. We seek rather to enrich him from his own internal sources. . . Such activity as this is pastoral work in the best sense of the word." (Freud, 1927, pp. 255-256) Much of what I have written may be regarded as a consequence of my effort to take Freud's foregoing view seriously. (Szasz, 1976, pp. 127-35)

Throughout his long life, Jung also struggled with the dilemma of whether to classify psychotherapy as a medical or as a religious enterprise. Although, as I showed, Jung too vacillated in his attitude toward this question, on the whole he assumed a more consistently antimedical and proreligious position on it than did Freud. (Szasz, 1978, pp. 158-75) In fact, the break between Freud and Jung, usually thought to center on their disagreement about the significance of sexuality in the etiology and therapy of the neuroses, lies much deeper, and is, I believe closely connected with the problem before us.

To put it simply, Freud was more ambitious and less honest about psychotherapy than Jung. Appraising the temper of his time correctly, Freud realized that the great legitimizer of the age was not religion but science. He insisted, therefore, that psychotherapy was a science, and he called his own version of it psychoanalysis.

Jung rejected such an opportunistic hitching of psychotherapy to the wagon of medical science. He maintained that religions were the forerunners of modern psychotherapies and that psychotherapeutic systems were actually ersatz religions. For example, in 1932 he writes: "In this matter (of spiritual needs) both the doctor and the patient deceive themselves. Although the theories of Freud and Adler come much nearer to getting at the bottom of the neuroses than does any earlier approach to the question from the side of medicine, they still fail, because of their exclusive concern with the drives, to satisfy the deeper spiritual needs of the patient. . .In a word, they do not give meaning enough to life. And it is only the meaningful that sets us free." (Jung, 1932, pp. 221-44, 1933, pp. 224-55)

"It is," Jung continues, "the priest or the clergyman, rather than the doctor, who should be most concerned with the problem of spiritual suffering. But in most cases the sufferer consults a doctor in the first place, because he supposes himself to be physically ill, and because certain neurotic symptoms can be at least alleviated by drugs." (Jung, 1932, p. 227) Jung concludes that "healing may be called a religious problem. . . .Religions are systems of healing for psychic illness. . . .That is why patients force the psychotherapist into the role of a priest, and expect and demand of him that he shall free them from their distress. That is why we psychotherapists must occupy ourselves with problems which, strictly speaking, belong to the theologians." (Jung, 1932, pp. 237, 241)

The problems Jung here highlights are still very much with us. Indeed, the positivistic--medical, psychological, and scientific--approach to the psychotherapies is today even more entrenched, concealed behind even thicker smoke screens of semantic and institutional legitimizations than it had been in 1933 when Jung wrote the following words:

> This Freudian father-complex, fanatically defended with such stubbornness and over-sensitivity, is a cloak for religiosity mis-understood; it is a mysticism expressed in terms of biology and the family relation. As For Freud's idea of the "super-ego", it is a furtive attempt to smuggle in his time-honored images of Jehovah in the dress of psychological theory. When one does things like that, it is better to say so openly. For my part, I prefer to call things by the

names under which they have always been
known. The wheel of history must not be
turned back, and man's advance towards a
spiritual. . .must not be denied. (Jung
1932, pp. 115-24)

Freud's declaration that the psychoanalyst is a
"secular pastoral worker" and that psychoanalysis is
"pastoral work in the best sense of the word," and
Jung's declaration that the psychotherapist occupies
the role of the priest and that the problems of psychotherapy "belongs to the theologians" have the most
far-reaching practical implications. They are comparable to the declarations, two hundred years ago,
of the abolitionists and Quakers that Negroes are
human beings. As the view that blacks are persons was
inconsistent with the institution of chattel slavery,
so the view that psychotherapy is religion is inconsistent with the institution of medical psychiatry.
Therein, precisely, lies both its threat and its promise.

In the New Testament, the words name and power
are synonymous. The power to name things, to classify
acts and actors, is the greatest power in the world.
Classifying "psychotherapies" and "psychotherapists"
thus reflects certain facts about the holders of
power. If we now classify certain forms of personal
conduct as illness, it is because most people believe
that the best way to deal with them is by responding
to them as if they were medical diseases. Similarly,
if we now classify certain other forms of personal conduct as psychotherapy, it is because most people believe that the best way to legitimize these activities
is by authenticating them as medical treatments.
(Szasz, 1970, Ch. 12)

Classifying human acts and actors is political,
because the classification will inevitably help some
persons and har others. Categorizing religion,
rhetoric, and repression as psychotherapy primarily
helps physicians and psychotherapists. If, however,
our aim in classifying psychotherapeutic interventions
is to help others--in particular those who want to
better understand the world they live in--then we shall
categorize such interventions as what they are--re-
ligion, rhetoric, and repression.

Language thus not only reveals and conceals acts

146

and actors; it also creates what and who they are. For example, in the first century A.D., Roman Christians were heretics; in the fourth century, they were possessors of the true faith. A few decades ago, oral-genital sex was a degrading perversion; now it is a delightful pastime. A few years ago, abortion was an abominable criminal act; now it is an accepted form of medical treatment. Obviously, it makes a great deal of difference to a great many people whether we call certain acts pastoral or psychotherapeutic, religious or medical.

The distinction between rhetoric and science was supremely important to Aristotle. The distinction between talking and treatment, spiritual caring and medical curing is equally important to anyone who wants to think clearly about such matters. As I showed, although some rhetoricians, such as Mesmer and Erb, claimed that their interventions were medical treatments, others, such as Freud and Jung, claimed that their interventions were both medical curings and spiritual carings. Such a dual claim has, indeed, continued to be advanced on behalf of psychiatry and psychotherapy by most of its propagandists. The fact that this claim has been accepted as valid by the intellectual, legal, and political authorities of most modern societies has had beneficial consequences for the claimants and baneful consequences for nearly everyone else. The result is that modern psychiatry and psychotherapy claim to be scientific religion or religious science, combining in a powerful alliance the forces of both religion and science. When that power is then allied with the modern state, the result is a fresh political force--a force at once arrogant and arbitrary, despotic and destructive.

My contention that all forms of psychotherapy comprise one or several elements of religion, rhetoric, and repression finds striking confirmation in the writings of Pierre Janet, one of the pioneers of modern medical psychotherapy. In his book, Psychological Healing, Janet considers the moral objections raised against suggestive therapy--especially that the hypnotist or suggestionist deceives his patient--and tries to refute them with the following argument: "I am sorry that I cannot share these exalted and beautiful scruples. . . My belief is that the patient wants a doctor who will cure; that the doctor's professional duty is to give any remedy that will be useful, and to prescribe it in the way in which it will do most good. Now I think that bread pills are medically indicated in certain cases and that they will act far more powerfully if I deck them out with impressive names. When I prescribe such a formidable placebo, I believe that I am fulfilling my professional duty." (Janet, 1925, Vol. II, p. 338)

The old rhetoric of partiotism is here transformed into the new rhetoric of therapeutism. The words and the imagery conjure up an irresistible justification, or so it seems to Janet. Who could object to a remedy that cures a sick patient? According to Janet, no one could, or should: "We are faced here with one of those conflicts between duties which are continually arising in practical life; and, for my part, I believe that the duty of curing my patient preponderates enormously over the trivial duty of giving him a scientific lecture which he would not understand and would have no use for." (Janet, 1925, Vol. II, p. 338)

Janet premises his claims on the tacit assumption that patients want to be lied to, that they want to infantilize themselves and paternalize their therapists. "There are some (patients)," he declares, "to whom, as a matter of strict moral obligation, we must lie." (Janet, 1925, Vol. II, p. 338) Why lying should be a matter or moral obligation on the part of a physician, Janet does not further explain. Perhaps, once more, he assumes as obvious that the doctor's relationship to his patient ought to be like that of a Platonic guardian to the citizen: the former "owes" it to the latter to pacify him with "noble lies". Thus does deception become the cornerstone of modern medical psychotherapeutics. Indeed, Janet explicitly asserts that hypnosis rests not only on deception but also on despotism, that is, on the domination of the subject by the hypnotist: "The relationship of a hypnotisable patient to a hypnotist does not differ in any essential way from the relationship of a lunatic to the superintendent of an asylum. By accepting this outlook, those who practice suggestion and hypnotism would escape a good many moral difficulties--difficulties which never trouble alienists". (Janet, 1925, p. 340) The ethical and political implications of this admission--namely, that hypnosis in particular and mad-doctoring in general depend on the pseudomedical tyrannization of the patient by the doctor--have been widely ignored. Thus, hypnosis enjoys periodic revivals as a "medical treatment" and the false analogy between chemical anesthesia and the so-called hypnotic trance persists.

Janet himself was, of course, an accomplished base rhetorician. For example, he tries to persuade the reader of the validity of his claims by pretending to be wholly empirical and therapeutic. "The only thing that really matters," he declares, "is that we should know whether hypnotism is practically effective. Have notable cures been achieved through hypnotic suggestion, employed in a definite fashion and to the exclusion of other methods? Generally speaking, the answer is in the affirmative." (Janet, 1925, p. 338) Like Freud, Janet dons the robes of the positivistic scientist and pronounces himself in possession of a scientific psychotherapy. Hence, to disagree with him is to deny science itself. "Hypnotic suggestion," asserts Janet, "is no longer a vague theriac. . . It is a definite treatment whose results can be ascertained. . .These characteristics (of hypnosis). . . enable us to emerge from the religious and moral epoch." (Janet, 1925, p. 367)

Hypnosis does indeed remain a useful model for exposing the true nature of all psychotherapies. It is the paradigm of ritualized repression and of medicalized mendacity, displaying, in a dramatically enacted form of personal pairing, both the faith and the folly that animate all attempts to transform the tragedies and triumphs of real life into the therapies of a fake science.

One of the most successful recent psychotherapeutic movements is Couéism or so-called autosuggestion. Its doctrine and practice illustrate dramatically the combination, in the concepts and claims of a modern psychotherapist, of the clerical cure of souls with the clinical treatment of minds.

Émile Coué (1857-1926) was a French pharmacist who became interested in the then-popular practice of hypnosis. At about the same time that Freud hit upon the idea that the royal road to the unconscious led through the analysis of dreams, Coué hit upon the idea

that the royal road to the unconscious led through the
analysis of dreams, Coué hit upon the idea that the
royal road to mental health led through the sufferer's
own inner self. The patient did not need to be hypno-
tized. He did not even need a therapist. The essential element in hypnotic "treatment" was the subject's
own resolution to recover from his "illness". Armed
with that idea, Coué instructed persons suffering
from nervous disorders to tell themselves--morning,
noon, and night,--that "every day and in every way I
am getting better and better." During the first two
decades of the twentiety century his popularity and
success were phenomenal. (Weatherhead, 1952, pp. 122-
28)

Instead of stressing interpretation and insight,
as Freud did, Coué emphasized resolution and ritual.
"Don't think of what you are saying," he told his
patients. "Say it as you say the litany in church."
(Weatherhead, 1952, p. 122) Freud demanded that the
patient "admit" that he is "ill" and promise to "free-
associate," that is, tell his analyst everything that
goes through his mind. Coué's rules of psychotherapy
were almost exactly the opposite. He insisted that
the patient not give a name to his alleged disease,
as if he had realized that such disorders were metaphorical in nature and acquired a literal existence
only through being named; and he insisted that the
patient articulate his resolve to recover in the present rather than in the future tense, as if he had
realized that decisions promised for future delivery
have no moral reality. Remarking on the magico-
religious character of modern psychotherapies, Leslie
Weatherhead offers this comment about Coué's method:
"It is strange, as one contemplates Coué's instructions
to a patient to repeat the words 'Ca passe' ('It will
pass') and to count the number of times he says those
words by fingering knots in a cord, to compare so
modern a direction with the practices of antiquity, in
which the magician untied a knot in a cord as he re-
cited each new spell". (Weatherhead, 1952, p. 22)

Coué had thus rediscovered an age-old wisdom--
namely, that when a respected authority instills faith
in a person and admonishes him to "get better" and
that when such a person places faith in the authority
and resolves to "recover" from an "illness" that consists largely or wholly of this having assumed the

sick role, then he is likely to derive a "therapeutic" benefit from the interaction and from his own attitudes and actions. The question is: How should such a simple and straightforward moral exhortation be categorized? Let us see how Coueists and modern psychotherapists classify it.

An English exposition of Coueism was published in 1922 by C. Harry Brooks. Entitled The Practice of Autosuggestion by the Method of Emile Coue, it includes a foreword by Coue himself. In keeping with the demands of the scientific age in which he was writing, Brooks declares that "autosuggestion is not a religion like Christian Science. . . It is a scientific method based on the discoveries of psychology." (Brooks, 1922, p. 47) Having unburdened himself of that ritual incantation required of the modern faith healer, Brooks is free to preach his, and Coue's faith: "Say it (the magic formula) with faith! You can only rob Induced Autosuggestion of its power in one way--by believing that it is powerless. . . The greater your faith, the more radical and the more rapid will be your results." (Brooks, 1922, p. 85)

In the concluding chapter of his book, Brooks reiterates that autosuggestion is both a science and a religion: "We should approach autosuggestion in the same reasonable manner as we approach any other scientific discovery." (Brooks, 1922, p. 114) But only six lines later, he declares: "Like religion, autosuggestion is a thing to practice. A man may be conversant with all the creeds in Christendom and be none the better for it; while some simple soul, loving God and his fellows, may combine the high principles of Christianity in his life without any acquaintance with theology. So it is with autosuggestion." (Brooks, 1922, pp. 114-115) To Coue and his followers, then, autosuggestion was at once a religious and a medical enterprise. They emphasized one or the other aspect of it, depending on the argument they wanted to put forward.

Actually, it would be difficult to imagine how anything could be more clearly a secular prayer for health than reciting Coue's formula. "Is not the affirmation contained in Coue's formula a kind of prayer?" asks Brooks, only to offer the standard denial of our age in reply to it: No it is not prayer but "a mere scientific technique!" (Brooks, 1922,

p. 119)

Although Coué was a pharmacist and hence a layman,
psychiatrists and psychiatric historians count him as
one of their own. For example, Alexander and
Selesnick, with their unflagging zeal for flattering
the medical profession, call Coué a "hypnotist, psychotherapist, and autosuggestionist" (Alexander and
Selesnick, p. 84)--despite the fact that Coue explicitly repudiated hypnotism. All this betokens still a-
nother aspect of the implacable resolve of psychotherapy to rob religion of as much as it can, and to
destroy what it cannot: contrition, confession,
prayer, faith, inner resolution, and countless other
elements are expropriated and renamed as psychotherapy;
whereas certain observances, rituals, taboos, and other
elements of religion are demeaned and destroyed as the
symptoms of neurotic or psychotic illnesses.

I submit that we ought to distinguish more sharply than is customary in contemporary medical, psychiatric, legal and political thought between language and
lesions, between lies and leukemia. My suggestion that
we separate medical from psychiatric interventions may
be countered with the assertion that persuasion constitutes an inseparable part of medical practice. For
example, physicians persuad diabetics to use insulin
and patients with cancer to submit to operations. Are
such medical recommendations, so this argument might
run, not an integral part of what we call "medical
treatment"? And if so, does not this fact contradict
the supposedly sharp demarcation between the physician's
prescription of drugs and surgical therapy and the
psychiatrist's prescription of drugs and psychotherapy?

The similarities between the prescriptive acts
of regular physicians and those of psychiatrists rests
on the same illusion as do the similarities between
the sick-role performances of bodily and mentally ill
patients. Both medical and mental patients usually
act as if they were sick. And both regular physicians
and psychiatrists usually act as if they were pre-
scribing treatments. To the extent that each of these
actors plays his role well--whether as patient or
doctor--his performance will be convincing; and to
that extend the demarcation between histopathology and
psychopathology, between medical and psychiatric treatment, may seem contrived or false. I have described
elsewhere the pretenses of neurotics and psychotics

claiming to be patients, but I have not heretofore
described the corresponding pretenses of psychiatrists
and psychotherapists claiming to be therapists.

What makes a physician a therapist? Certainly
not the mere fact that he is a physician. Not all
physicians treat patients and not all are therapists.
Pathologists and diagnostic radiologists, to name
only two obvious examples, do not treat patients and
are not therapists. What makes a physician a therapist is that he performs a physiochemical act on the
patient's body that is, or is considered, therapeutic.
A pathologist or radiologist may recommend the removal of a tumor; but such an act is not a form of
therapy. Only the removal of the tumor is. In the
course of medical treatment the physician may use
persuasion as a part of, or preliminary to, his actual
therapeutic performance; but persuasion is not, in
itself, a form of medical treatment.

Psychiatric treatment differs from this, and it
does so in different ways in the so-called somatic
therapies and the psychotherapies. Somatic therapies--
for example, the use of drugs or shock or lobotomy--
involve the employment of physiochemical interventions
on the patient's body. But since the intervention is
not aimed at any demonstrable pathological lesion, but
on the contrary is aimed at the patient's undesirable
behavior, it is wrong to classify it as therapy.
Poisoning and electrocuting criminals are, after all,
also physiochemical interventions on human bodies.
But since the subjects are not patients, we do not
call these procedures treatment.

In psychotherapy the situation is altogether
different from that obtained in regular medical
therapy. Psychotherapy, as I have shown, is religion
or rhetoric (or repression, a contingency about which
I shall say no more here). The result of psychotherapy
can thus only be that the subject is, or is not, converted or persuaded to feel, think, or act differently
than has been his habit. The "patient" changes some
of his ways; or he remains the same. The psychotherapist does not do anything but talk. If there is
any change in the "patient", it is, in the last analysis, brought about by the "patient" himself. Hence,
it is false to say that the psychotherapist treats
or is a therapist. It would be more accurate to say

153

that the "patient" in psychotherapy treats or is a
therapist, because he treats himself. But that, too,
would be using the term treatment metaphorically,
inasmuch as such a person treats himself only in the
sense in which any person who submits himself to an
activity cooperates with athletic, education, or religious influence or instruction treats himself.

Still, physicians and patients insist that psychotherapy is medical treatment. This is no more
surprising than that Medieval Catholic priests insisted that ceremonial wine is human blood. Such a
confusion and conflation of ceremonial and scientific
concepts and performances is rarely accidental. In
the case of the Eucharist, the mythologized category
error was an integral part of Medieval Christian
theology; in the case of psychotherapy, it is an integral part of modern medical theology. In medicine,
and especially in psychiatry, the clear distinction
between science and religion, so typical of contemporary thought, is obscured. In the natural sciences,
we distinguish between astrology and astronomy,
alchemy and chemistry. But in medicine we do not
distinguish--often we are officially forbidden to
distinguish between healing by spiritual and moral influences on the one hand, and by chemical and physical
interventions on the other. It is, of course, mainly
through psychiatry, and its core concepts of mental
illness and psychotherapy, that the distinction between
the cure of bodies and the cure of souls is confused,
condemned, and cast out of official science.

Whether we classify religion, rhetoric, and repression as psychotherapy, or vice versa, has, of
course the most obvious and far-reaching practical implications. Religion (morals and ritual), rhetoric
(speech and gestures), and repression, (constraint
and punishment) are all matters of the utmost concern
to every legal and political system, especially to
the American legal and political system where the
precise sphere of action of each--particularly their
freedom from government interference and their exclusion from government support--is clearly defined.

There is, however, no comparable definition of
the proper sphere of the state with respect to medical
matters. Insofar as the role of the state in relation
to health is examined and articulated, it is usually

in the spirit of naïve medicalism, reflecting the
false premise that in the area of treatment, unlike
that of salvation, there are no fundamental conflicts
between the individual and the state. As a result,
the most varied interests have sought, in the name of
health, to enlist the support of the modern state.
They have all succeeded. For example, we saw how
Heinroth based his whole psychiatric program on the
premise that the financial support and legal imposition
of mental treatment were the self-evident duties of
the state. Since then, the idea that the preservation
and promotion of health are obligations the government
owes to its citizens has become, the whole world over,
an article of faith compared to which the Medieval
belief in Christianity is veritable skepticism.

As a result, most people now believe that it is
a good thing that the state defines what is sickness
and what is treatment and that the state pays for
whatever treatment people need. What most people do
not understand, indeed seem disinclined to understand,
is that the state may, and therefore will, define as
sickness whatever the people might want to do for
themselves; that it may, and therefore will, define
as treatment whatever the government might want to do
to the people; and that it may, and therefore will,
tax the people for "medical" services that range from
denying Laetrile to those persons who want it to im-
posing psychiatric imprisonment on those who do not
want it. Clearly, the future scope of such "service"
promises to include an array of therapeutic pro-
hibitions and prescriptions of truly Orwellian pro-
portions.

THEOLOGY AND PSYCHOLOGY:
A HUMANISTIC PERSPECTIVE

Joseph E. Morris

Within recent years the dialogue between psychologists and theologians has been steadily increasing, enhanced by the emergence of humnaistic psychology and the holistic health movement. The subjective methodology and phenomenological epistemology of the existentialist/humanist approach offers more flexibility than other psychological viewpoints and focuses on areas of interest to theologians: self-growth, values, inter-personal relations, self-actualization, and creativity. The integrative philosophy of the holistic health movement has heightened sensitivity to the need for cooperative dialogue between disciplines whose purpose is the improvement of the human condition, including theology and psychology.

A number of prominent psychologists have engaged in cooperative inquiry with theology, including Gordon Allport (1950, 1955), W.H. Clark (1958, 1967), and Abraham Maslow (1954, 1964), making significant contributions toward a reconciliation of the two disciplines. From the theological side Paul Tillich (1951, 1952, 1958) has emphasized the existential meanings for the theory and practice of psychology. Borrowing from Tillich's definition of religion, the study of man's "ultimate concern," Joseph Royce (1962, 1967) has formulated a metaphoristic approach which embraces concepts common to existentialism, theology, and psychology.

The dialogue between psychology and theology received an added boost in the early 1960's when an APA committee was established to study the fundamental presuppositions of the two disciplines. The efforts of that committee, which extended over a three and one-half year period, resulted in Joseph Havens' _Psychology and Religion_ (1968), a series of structured reflections including actual dialogue between participants.

Few would argue that formal dialogue is occuring between theology and psychology. This cooperative experience on the formal, theoretical level, into the

157

operational level of applied therapy, has apparently
not yet had its impact on the grass roots level of
day-to-day, secular therapy. The conflict was
recently manifested by Paul Clement (APA Monitor,
June, 1978) in his charge that "American psychology
has consistently discriminated against organized religion" (p. 2). There are many who would agree with
his contention. In a current edition of APA Monitor
(November, 1981) only two journals (Journal of Psychology and Judaism and Pastoral Psychology) indicated
theological content out of a considerable number of
APA journals, suggesting that the professional
heirarchy attaches a limited value to the role of
theology in emotional and mental health.

Clement's statements appear too polemical and
general, but he does raise a pertinent and glaring
issue. There is a mood today in some quarters of
professional psychology which shuns association with
theological themes and symbols of Western culture.
This air of "guilt by dis-association" on the part of
some is both unnecessary and unfortunate.

Organized religion must be held accountable for
some of the lack of dialogue with psychology. Un-
essential programs, irrelevant messages, self-right-
eous excesses, and contradictory behavior have caused
large segments of our society, not just psychologists,
to look to the role of religious institutions with
reserve and skepticism. Though many theologians are
aware of these negative factors, their earnest
attempts to understand humanity realistically "have
been eclipsed by mythologies, christologies, Judaic-
Hellenistic metaphysics and dogmatics which bear little
resemblance to contemporary personal delimmas and
problems" (Morris, 1980, p. 93). This in no way implies that myths, symbols, and metaphysics have
nothing to do with theology. It is to say, however,
that when these applications fail to struggle with
the core issues of day-to-day living, they become
powerless and are thus appropriately jettisoned from
the mainstream of theological discourse.

Psychologists are not blameless in regards to
the split with some of their counterparts in the
world of theology. In the name of science, some
psychological positions reject documentation of any
phenomena or experiences not verifiable or validated

through empirical means. This narrow positivistic approach has repelled some theologians who might otherwise seek active and cooperative dialogue.

Realistically, psychologists and theologians, mental health therapists and pastoral counselors cannot afford to exclude each other mutually from their therapeutic domains. They share common goals and concerns. An avant' garde therapist working with a Southern Baptist fundamentalist must be willing to accept that his therapeutic goal is

> not a summum bonum; it is only one goal among many. The religious person may choose the living out of a high ethic, or the nurturing of spiritual experience at the expense of some values of mental health. (Havens, 1968, p. 104)

Conflicting cultural values should not preclude unconditional positive regard and empathy, though that is often the case. Humane therapy participates with individuals openly, accepting them within their cultural context, which might mean red-clay, "bible-thumping," pentecostalism. Here is the rub. Counselor integrity can also not be sacrificed. An honest, empathic relationship does have its limits.

It is not the therapist's role, from a humanistic viewpoint, to deprecate, alter, or attempt to destroy a client's religious orientation, one he or she has held since childhood. It is, however, the therapist's function "to create an atmosphere in which the client's defensive reactions are reduced, thus precluding narrow, selective perceptions and allowing for a greater participation in reality" (Morris, 1980, p.94). Vaughn (1965) suggests this means encouraging religious individuals to become more open to other religious realities and concepts, enabling them to choose freely what they in fact do believe in a way which is very real to them. The problem with many religiously oriented clients is their inability to articulate what they do believe in a way that implies ownership of their belief.

It is difficult for constructive dialogue to occur without some common hermeneutics, in our case, keys for interpreting the meanings of human existence. Traditional attempts have tended to flounder

around the ongoing debate between empiricism and
rationalism, which in one guise or another, is the
nature of the current conflict between some schools
of psychology and theology. Royce (1962, 1967) has
provided an alternative epistemology, namely meta-
phorism. Through this approach, the underlying psychological processes of reality are seen as "symbolic"
and "intuitive."

> ...all forms of knowledge, the sciences,
> the humanities, the arts, are symbolic
> manifestations of man's cultural evolution,
> and that the history of the development
> of the human psyche lies symbolically
> hidden in the major myths of mankind. (p.8)

Carlton Berenda (1957) drew a similar perspective
when he stated that the Bible and "the writings of
the great mystics and religions of India" offer "a
very rich source of relevant raw material and
theoretical insights for the clinician" (quoted in
Havens, 1968, p. 34).

The meaning of existence is conveyed through
words, symbols which point to our Lebenswelt, felt
meanings of lived experience. Both religious and
psychological language are concerned with the gut
issues of life, the questions of meaning, security,
frustration, and hopes: "Who am I?" "What is my
origin?" "What should I become and be?" "What is
of value?" "What is the meaning and future destiny
of my life and the history in which it participates?"
"How can I be whole again?" "What is the meaning of
my death?" Whether labeled existential or "ultimate
concern," when we ask questions we have entered the
overlapping pursuits and inquiries of both psychology
and theology.

> When we come to understand that the meanings
> behind and under the symbols share an exis-
> tential ultimacy, we have established a
> basis for useful and purposeful dialogue
> between therapists and clerics, between
> non-religious and religious counselors.
> (Morris, 1980, p. 95)

Religious language today is criticized, justi-
fiably so, as cumbersome and irrelevant, its myths

160

and symbols no longer reflecting those basic issues
of existence which once caused them to vibrate with
life and meaning. Pregoff (1953) reflected on this
current state of theological language:

> To say that an individual has "faith" is
> to say, psychologically, that he can live
> his symbols, that they are alive for him;
> and to say that an individual is "skeptical"
> means that the symbols are no longer spon-
> taneously active or alive within him.
> (pp. 209-210)

The same could be said of some psychological language.

Psychologists and theologians are concerned
with the same issue in their attempts to extract
meaning from an existence which is constantly evolving. The differences seem to be primarily linguistic.
Beneath the superficial trappings of the languages
lies a shared fundamental language of being, which
moves behind and under the word symbols and myths.
This assumption provides a basis for more than just
dialogue and rapprochement between psychologists and
theologians. It is a framework within which a
cooperative, working relationship can gel and grow as
the two disciplines pursue their common goal of the
whole, healthy personality.

A review of Judaeo-Christian themes and symbols
will reveal significant parallels with the basic
concepts of humanistic psychology. Both reflect
similar understandings of human nature and what constitutes the healthy personality. I will not attempt
to deal with major differences which exist between
religion and scientific psychology simply because they
exceed the scope of this discussion. I have also
attempted to steer clear of theoretical arguments
pertaining to the various positions of both religious
and non-religious psychologists.

Basic Concepts of Humanistic Psychology

Humanistic psychology has been criticized for
being amorphorus and diffuse to the extent that no
clear boundaries or limits are identifiable. In a
major statement, Wertheimer (1978) said of humanistic
psychology: "There is little agreement about an

explicit meaning of the phrase, which typically is used in a very vague manner" (p. 739). Wertheimer and others make some valid claims about the eclectic nature of humanistic psychology, but the claim that there "is little agreement about an explicit meaning of the phrase" is not a just assessment of the movement today.

A consensus of theoretical concepts has been emerging since the First International Congress of Humanistic Psychology in August of 1970. Charlotte Bühler, president of that first conference, was responsible for providing some shape to these themes and further defined them in conjunction with Melanie Allen (1972). In an earlier chapter in this volume I have condensed those concepts, drawing from the writings of other prominent humanists as Carl Rogers, J.F.T. Bugental, Rollo May, Abraham Maslow, Adrian Van Kaam, and Sidney Jourard, to mention a few (Cf. also Morris, 1979):

1. Emphasis upon the whole person as a model, importance of the individual self, and the uniqueness of persons.
2. A positive theoretical model of persons as active, free, and responsible.
3. A theory of knowledge based upon immediate experience.
4. The self as a central core system of personality; intentionality as basic to self-discovery.
5. Values oriented to life goals; self-actualization; and self-transcendence.
6. Creativity as a universal human characteristic.

Comparison with Biblical Themes

The whole person and individuality. A fundamental premise of humanistic psychology is the understanding of the whole as being greater than the sum of its parts and that "the central core of personality consists in its unity and uniqueness" (Severin, 1965, p. 3). Maslow (1965) summarized this viewpoint:

Many psychologists are content to work with but a portion of human being, indeed making a virtue out of such limitation. They forget

that their task ultimately is to give us a unified, empirically based concept of the whole
human being....(p. 23)

The Judaeo-Christian understanding of humanity
is similar. Personhood implies the whole person.
Body, mind, and soul are unified, not sliced into
compartments which function independently of each
other. The Hebrew word for body, nephesh, means
literally a union of body, mind, and spirit. The New
Testament word for body, soma, means the same, reflecting upon the totality of personhood. Curran (1968)
suggests that "one of the central tendencies of our
Judaeo-Christian culture is to regard man as caught
midway in a complex mosaic of spirit and flesh, of
knowing and feeling--and to consider the pursuit of
self-knowledge basic to self-development and personal
fulfillment" (in Havens, p. 98). The early influences
of Hellenistic dualism and later perversions of
Puritanism have been largely responsible for the dis-
tortion of this basic biblical understanding of personality.

Much more than being a treatise on God, the Bible
is an unfolding drama about people, individuals with
their personal conflicts and frustrations. Even the
heros, the super-humans (eg. Moses, Noah, Joseph,
Samson, Gideon, etc.) manifest their doubts and
frailties despite the epic grandness in which they are
portrayed. The book of Job may well be one of the
most humanistic testimonies in literary history. The
Psalms, cannonized rather late in Jewish history, place
an even heavier emphasis upon individualism than was
common in their times.

The human dimension is prominent in the New
Testament. From one perspective, the stories and
letters deal more with universal human conflicts than
with the Christ, though he is the focal point. When
examined closely, as some contemporary theologians
have done, the scriptures yield a clearer picture of
the humanness of Jesus of Nazareth rather than his
divinity heavily attributed to the Christ figure by the
later church. Contrary to the claims of many, the New
Testament does not project an ideal person which one
should become. The statement attributed to Jesus "to
be ye therefore perfect..." is an unfortunate mis-
translation. The Greek word for perfect, teleios,

163

does not imply perfect in the sense of the Greek ideal, but it denotes "complete," "whole." The interpretation could equally and more accurately read, "Be a whole person."

The concept of grace in both testaments is interpreted by most orthodox theologians to mean divine acceptance of humans as well as personal self-acceptance of others. Authentic being and self-expression, congruence, are central themes. People were called to "be themselves." This concept is implicit in the word "Yahweh," the Hebrew word for God, which translated means "I am who I am." The teachings and actions of Jesus are characterized as expressions of this dominant biblical theme. Humans are not made for the sake of religious institutions and traditions, but religious faith's purpose is to help people experience the freedom of being their true selves. "Man was not made for the Sabbath, the Sabbath was made for man." Through sayings such as this and with his use of the parable (unique in Jewish literature), Jesus launched a sharp attack on the organized religion of his own time which in itself was de-humanizing and impersonal.

Positive, free and responsible humanity. Humanistic psychologists see humans as active mediators of their own existence. Humans exist in a perpetual state of freedom, psychologically speaking. This is fundamental to their humanistic understanding of the nature of humanity. There can be no possibility of "self-becoming" without the pre-condition of freedom. We are free to become what we choose. Or in the words of Jean-Paul Sartre, "we become our choices." Rollo May (1961) adds, "within the limits of our given world" (p. 13). Individuals are responsible for, must answer for, their decisions. This understanding of responsibility allows them to become free moral agents.

The debate among theologians between individual free will and divine omnipotent control has raged for centuries and is not likely to subside. Most ecclesiastical doctrines promote an ambiguous "will of God" which diminishes human freedom, in some cases eliminating it all together. Unfortunately, they can find exegetical support in some biblical passages. But if one considers the larger context of the biblical tradition, humans are viewed from the eyes of an unconditional, positive regarding God. Despite the unfortunate doctrine of original sin, the Jewish-Christian "doctrine of man" advocates equally for the potential for good within human nature. The choices are left to individuals.

The Websters New World Dictionary (1960) defines a humanist as "one whose belief consists of faith in man and devotion to human well-being" (p. 1212). Based on this definition, the God of the Jewish-Christian heritage could well be the first humanist. What God is recorded as creating "is good, is very good." From the beginning a theme of basic trust is present. The events recorded in the Old Testament narrative are placed in the hands of humans by a God of patience rather than by a God of manipulation: "Be fruitful and multiply, and fill the earth and subdue it; and have dominion..." (Genesis 1:28, King James Version).

Responsibility was also expected as a result of the investment of trust. In the creation myth Adam and Eve were entrusted with responsibility and given choice. The results of their choices were consequences they had to own. Existentially, the story of Adam and Eve is the story of every man and woman. No deus ex machina swung from the wings like some Greek god to rescue them. Unmistakably, the biblical record does refer to those miraculous events when God intervened on behalf of "his people." But more realistically, and with greater impact, the record recalls unabashedly the absence of God, the crucifixion being the ultimate confirmation of that absence. More often than not, people were left to their own decisions and choices. "They were free to 'go to hell,' to choose who they were, what their attitude would be toward the things which happened to them, in essence, to choose their own version of humanity" (Morris, 1980, pp. 98-99).

Jesus is personified no differently in the New Testament. He was a "question man," not an "answer man," a confronter as much, if not more, than he was a rescuer. The literature portryas him as returning others' questions to themselves, encouraging self-examination and the experiential ownership of answers. He is described, in near Rogerian fashion, as

accepting others unconditionally, unmasking preten-
sions, and extending a confidence and openness which
gave them permission to express themselves spontaneously and authentically. He sought authentic
decisions from those he challenged and confronted.
The record reflects a near total absence of coersion,
pressure, or manipulation. Those whom he encountered
were offered the freedom to become who they were, and
challenged to bear the responsibility of their choices.

Knowledge as experiential relationship with reality.

Two basic principles provide the basis for
humanistic epistemology: (1) experience is the only
trustworthy condition for self-knowledge, and (2)
reality can be known only experientially through
participation in it: "There is no such thing as
truth of reality for a living human being except as he
participates in it, is conscious of it, and has some
relationship to it" (May, 1961, p. 14).

The Judaeo-Christian literary tradition is clear
about religious knowledge. It must be experienced to
possess any validity for self or others. Of great
significance is the fact that the Hebrew word for
knowledge, yada, is the equivalent of their expression
for sexual intercourse. The two are used inter-
changeably throughout the Old Testament. To "Be still
and know that he is God..." is to share in the ultimate intimacy. The nature of this intimate encounter
became the basis for Martin Buber's (1958) I and Thou,
a popular handbook for both theologians and psychologists. The theme of experiential knowledge pervades
New Testament content as well. Having experienced the
Christ event is fundamental for apostleship in the
developing church. St. Paul's credentials are suspect
because of the doubts some had about his "experience."
At the interpersonal level, only as individuals
experience themselves are they able to relate meaning-
fully to others.

The self and intentionality.

For humanistic
psychologists the self is the "core system" of personality and human behavior, the source of individual goal
setting. May (1961) calls the self "the cneter at

Which I know myself as the one responding" (pp. 34-35);
Allport (1961) refers to it as "some kind of core in
our being" (p. 110); and Bugental describes self as
"irreducibly a unity...the essential being" (pp. 201-
202). The "core self" and the concept of intentionality
are inseparable. In reference to intentionality May
(1965) states the "power to take some stand" is the
"never-lost kernel" of one's existence; it is the
capacity by which we constitute meanings in life"
(pp. 203). Humans demonstrate intentionality in the
decisions they make. Through the ownership of decisions and choices, identity grows, consciousness of
self intensifies. Bugental(1965)referred to intentionality as the basis upon which identity is built.

It is perhaps on the related themes of self and
intentionality that Jewish-Christian anthropology
draws closest to the core of the humanistic dynamic.
Earlier the Hebrew interpretation of Yahweh, the
God-head, was given: "I am who I am." The same word
can as well be translated "I cause to be what I cause
to be." Yahweh, God, is the one who causes things to
be and to happen. At the highest level identity and
intentionality are incorporated. The creation of
humans in the "image of God" moves the logic one step
further to the plane of finite behavior: "We are
who we are and we cause to be what we cause to be."
In the biblical context this understanding is related
to the ethic of love. Individuals are not capable
of expressing genuine love, agape, toward others unless
they can genuinely accept and love themselves. "Love
thy neighbor as thyself" is a profound psychological
statement pointing to genuine self-respect, a
positive self concept as the basis for altruistic
behavior. Kierkegaard, Tillich, Buber and other
theologians with psychological orientation have
stressed this theme. Self-identity emerges through the
crucible of decision. Tillich (1952) stated that the
individual becomes human only at the point of decision.
Self-respect and intentionality are conditional for
the biblical understanding of the healthy, integrated,
whole personality. Indeed, the word holy itself
stems from the Greek holos, meaning whole.

Endgoals and creativity. An expression of the
free, responsible, intentional self is goal-directed
behavior. The ultimate achievement, or endgoal,

167

proposed by some within the humanistic movement is "self-realization" or "self-actualization." Viktor Frankl (1969) called it "self-transcendence...a constructive characteristic of being human that always points and is directed to something other than itself" (p. 113). The difference in terminology appears more semantical than qualitative. The common denominator for all of these expressions is living with a sense of purpose and direction, applying one's creativity in an open, non-determined future: "Only the flexibly creative person can really manage the future, only the one who can face novelty with confidence and without fear" (Maslow, 1961, p. 56).

Judaeo-Christian teleology, the study of ultimate purposes, is heavily laden with otherworldly content. However, temporal teleological themes abound as well, especially those emphasizing altruistic behavior, the love of others as the ultimate expression of divine presence and fulfillment. As indicated above, these themes run parallel with the goals of humanistic psychology, namely, the enrichment of interpersonal relationships and the creative, open involvement of people with each other.

Conclusion

It was not the intent of this study to prove the convergence of psychological and religious fundamentals. However, it can be justly said that they are not dichotomous, but "lie along a continuum defined by degrees of preciseness of conceptualization and verification" (Havens, 1968, p. 88). The relationship between religion and psychology can be, and is, characterized in a variety of ways by theorists and practitioners from both disciplines. The attempt in this article was to show how common symbols and linguistic expressions can provide a basis for increased dialogue and research and how humanistic psychology is proving itself to be an appropriate and adequate forum for those advancements. It is important for rigorous scientific research to expand its epistemology to include the intuitive with the empirical dimension, giving legitimacy to the former as a valid field of inquiry.

At the more practical, grassroots level, non-religious and religious oriented therapists need not split blindly over issues which have so much in common. Many basic conflicts and differences remain. But a recognizable bridge is available "for an intellectual empathy if not a genuine affective, empathic understanding of the client's religious conflicts and/or emotional stresses caused by religious variables" (Morris, 1980, p. 101).

PSYCHOTHERAPY: WHATEVER BECAME OF ORIGINAL SIN?

Roger J. Sullivan

Moral philosophy, as it often is understood and practiced today, consists in a careful analysis of the uses of and logical interrelationships between key concepts in moral language. One purpose of such an analysis is to attain more clarity than we usually have about morality and moral claims.

The analytic method also can be used to examine moral theories and to compare them with one another. Comparing moral theories can help us appreciate, for example, how enormously moral theorizing is influenced by the views a person takes about the nature of human nature. Aristotle and Kant, for instance, each began with a different conception of what it is to be a human being: Aristotle with a naturalistic and humanistic view, and Kant with a traditional Christian view. As a consequence, each developed different and incompatible conceptions about the character of the morally best person and about the process of moral development and education (Sullivan, 1974).[1]

It seems to me that many of the contrasts which obtain between Aristotle and Kant also hold when we compare much of contemporary psychotherapy, which explicitly or implicitly presupposes a naturalistic, humanistic view of human nature, with traditional, orthodox Christianity, in which the predominant conception of human nature is at least very similar to Kant's. What makes such a comparison interesting is the fact that so many pastoral counselors today use psychotherapeutic methods and adopt psychotherapeutic goals.

In this paper I will argue that any alliance between traditional Christianity and humanistic psychotherapy is an uneasy union, due for reappraisal. For

---

[1]An article (1974) in which I compared aspects of the moral theories of Aristotle and Kant has generated several other articles in the journals as well as an N.E.H. Summer Seminar.

despite contemporary theological reassessments of
Christian doctrines and despite differences between
denominational interpretations of those doctrines,
there still are questions about whether doctrinal beliefs held by the vast majority of Christians today
and the humanistic philosophy permeating most psychotherapies today can be made compatible with each other.

To show the force of these questions, I will contrast a "standard" Christian view of human nature,
most explicitly found in the Pauline writings, with
the comparable view presupposed by one such kind of
psychotherapy familiar to pastoral counselors, Transactional Analysis. Transactional Analysis admirably
exhibits several fundamental characteristics shared
by all contemporary humanistic psychotherapies. It is
completely naturalistic in its explanations of human
behavior; it also is thoroughly empirical in nature.
Because it takes the view that present behavior is ex-
plicable only in terms of preceding causal determinants,
it regards present behavior as mainly the product of
past experiences, particularly those in early childhood. The origin of dysfunctional behavior, therefore,
is to be found in malefic (particularly parental) influences.

These same views can be found in the writings of
such authors as Abraham Maslow, Albert Ellis, Erich
Fromm, Carl Rogers, and Gordon Allport. There is,
however, this important difference. Transactional
Analysis (as I will shortly argue) minimally presumes
only that basic human nature is neutral, that is,
initially neither psychologically healthy nor unhealthy, while others make the more optimistic claim
that the human person is basically good, born with a
natural internal harmony and capacity for making good
personal decisions. The implication will be that, if
any form of humanistic psychotherapeutic theory can be
compatible with traditional Christian belief, it will
be Transactional Analysis; and if it turns out to be
conceptually irreconcilable with traditional Christian
belief, then clearly other, stronger forms of humanistic theories cannot be compatible with traditional
Christian belief.

In the following two sections I will set out first
the traditional Christian view of man and then the
view   I   think is presupposed in Transactional

Analysis. In the third section I will point out conceptual difficulties between the two views, and in the next sections I will summarize three efforts to solve those problems. The final section will consist of a brief conclusion.

I.

At the very heart of traditional Christian belief is the doctrine of the redemption--the doctrine that God sent his own Son to save mankind. This doctrine presupposes that man is in need of some such divine intervention, and this need is explained by another fundamental Christian doctrine, the doctrine of original sin. These two doctrines frequently appear together in the New Testament: "As one man's trespass led to condemnation for all men" (Rom. 5:18), and, "As in Adam all die, so also in Christ shall all be made alive" (1 Cor. 15:20).

Denominations and theologians differ about how to interpret the account of the fall in Genesis. Some interpret it literally, as describing an historical event; others interpret it as a religious myth. Some hold for monogenism, others for polygenism. Some say man's sinful nature is inherited from Adam; others, like Niebuhr (1964), say Adam represents the universal human condition. Nonetheless, major denominations agree that all human beings are sons and daughters of Adam. Minimally, this means (1) that man, who originally was created by God as good, in His own image, destined to live in intimacy with God, now is born into a condition of deprivation, a state of alienation from God, possessing a wounded, scarred (and some say totally depraved) nature: and (2) that each person is born a sinner, both in tendency and in inevitable fact (see Rom. 3:23, 5:12). This is the "propensity for evil" which the Christian philosopher Immanuel Kant (1973) described as universal, radical, innate, and inextirpable.

Church literature is filled with references to this doctrine. Article IX of The Book of Common Prayer (1928, p. 604), for example, speaks of "the fault and corruption of the Nature of every man, that naturally is engendered of the offspring of Adam; whereby man is. . . of his own nature inclined to evil." Moreover, following the practice of the early church,

173

most worship services today include a public and communal confession of guilt for sin; and a good deal of preaching is aimed at impressing upon congregations the fact that they are sinners who may not feel as much guilt for their sins as they should.

According to this doctrine, we sin because our nature is irrevocably flawed, and we find ourselves subject to constant internal disharmony or moral conflict. No one has described the nature of this spiritual struggle more poignantly than St. Paul in the famous passage where he wrote: "I do not understand my own actions. For I do not do what I want, but I do the very thing I hate. . . . I can will what is right, but I cannot do it. . . . Now if I do what I do not want, it is no longer I that do it, but sin which dwells within me" (Rom. 7:15-20).

According to this religious tradition, a person cannot by himself overcome his estrangement from and be reconciled to God; only God's saving grace can restore a person to the original relationship of love. This is the meaning of Jesus' salvific suffering and death (see Matt. 26:28; John 3:16-17; 1 Cor. 15:45). But, as the Apostle Paul learned, even after conversion human nature remains irrevocably maimed, and Christians are not relieved of their continuing internal moral struggle, their propensity to sin.Consequently, living as a Christian means involvement in a process, never completed, in which the individual, now suspended between sin and redemption, struggles to transcend his sinful nature and increasingly to relate himself to God (Tillich, 1963). He still finds he cannot help but sin, yet he still remains responsible for his sins, for none occur necessarily. Consequently, the Christian remains utterly dependent on the continuing grace of God to forgive him and to sustain the process of sanctification.

Let me summarize now this view of what it is to be a human being. (1) Although there is no attempt to discount the influence of malevolent external agencies, the fundamental locus for the problem of evil (sin) is within the individual person: we are all born with a nature at war with itself, and we cannot alter our nature. (2) We can, however, work to subdue our rebellious nature, but only with the help of God. (3) The conceptual connection between the

174

doctrine of original sin on the one hand and the doctrines of redemption and grace on the other is so close that it is not possible to thin the meaning of the first without also radically weakening the meaning of the others.

II.

Transactional Analysis is both a psychological theory and a psychotherapeutic method (James, 1971). Although it is a relatively young school, its theory stands within a long Western tradition of humanistic and naturalistic thought that can be traced back at least to Aristotle. Both Aristotle and Eric Berne, the founder of TA, were methodological empiricists; both developed their views about the structure and development of human beings on the basis of their observations. This is to be expected, since Aristotle first was trained as a biologist and botanist and Berne as a physician.

Both Aristotle and Berne decided that it is a drastic mistake to think of a person only as an individual; we are social in nature, and our internal psychic life is formed by the ways others have transacted with us and we have learned to transact with others. Both men consequently placed enormous stress on the influence of those responsible for a child's nuturing. Human nature is, within limits, plastic, and a person's feelings about himself and others all are learned from his relationships with others. Conflicts with others tend to generate internal conflicts which in turn tend to exhibit themselves in estrangements from others. Likewise, the person who has been taught to accept and love himself is in the best position to accept and love others. Aristotle described the developmental process under the rubric of character-formation and Berne under the rubric of script-formation (Sullivan, 1977; Berne, 1972).

Berne and his followers avoid saying anything about the nature of the child before the developmental process begins, and in one place Berne explicitly eschewed any attempt "to deal, formally at least, with the essence of being, the Self" (Berne, 1972, p. 396). But since he agreed with Aristotle in regarding present behavior as the product of past experiences, the view of human nature implicitly present in TA theory

175

must be very much like that explicitly set forth by Aristotle.

Unaffected by the later Christian view of human nature, Aristotle took the position that the newly born and normally endowed human infant begins life from a morally and psychologically neutral position. Moral goodness, he wrote, "is implanted in us neither by nature nor contrary to nature. . . . We do not by nature develop into good or evil men" (<u>Eth. Nic.</u> 3.5. 1114a31-b11). What a child does have at birth, he thought, are various potentialities; they are "capacities for opposites," because they can be developed in either psychologically healthy or unhealthy ways, in either morally good or evil ways. According to Aristotle, a child's emotions are neither good nor bad, but they are "wild" and "undisciplined" and need to be guided and shaped by his tutors. Although a child may be born genetically defective or may be adversely traumatized, Aristotle believed that generally the process of developing and shaping of personality is accomplished by habituation.

The Aristotelianism tacitly underlying TA theory, therefore, expects the developmental process to involve some conflicts with parental figures as a child is taught emotional control. It is not surprising, then, that a child typically assumes, in TA terminology, an "I'm not OK, You are" position. But this need not be more than a stage in normal growth. Internal conflicts (between different parts of the soul for Aristotle or between ego-states for TA) which persist into chronological maturity are not inevitable but can be traced to defective developmental experiences which have been internalized and which are replayed, often repetitiously (Berne, 1972, pp. 31-109). However common they may be, such internal psychic conflicts are not the norm; they are not an ineluctable part of what it is to be a human being.

Both Aristotle and Berne concede that individual adults may resist doing what they need to do to reach the ideal in personality development. Aristotle admits that often desirable behavior may be all that can be obtained, and Berne, who has a more sophisticated theory, allows that therapeutic treatment may succeed only in achieving symptomatic control or relief rather than a cure of internal conflicts. Perhaps no one ever totally achieves complete

integration (Berne, 1972, p. 396). Yet, for both
Aristotle and Berne, the ideal and norm toward which
we are to aim is the autonomous adult who has achieved
and who enjoys substantial internal integrity (or
integration), in which reason (or the Adult ego-state)
acts as the "executive" of social control, determining
what kind of emotions and what kind of conduct are
appropriate in each kind of situation. Such a person
does not have to expend enormous energy keeping himself (his Parent and Child ego-states) under control,
for he already _is_ is a self-controlled, self-directed
person. In Aristotelian terms, his character is so
formed that he is committed to living rightly and well,
and he feels very good about doing so; in TA terms,
he operates from an "I'm OK, You're OK" life position.

Some of my readers may protest the identification
of Berne as Aristotelian, because Aristotle usually
did not distinguish between psychological and moral
health (and illness) while Berne generally avoided
both the use of specifically moral categories and
any discussion about how psychological and moral
categories might be answered depends, of course, to a
great extent on how one defines the nature of morality.)
In one of his earlier works Berne suggested that the
Adult ego-state might have "ethical aspects" (Berne,
1961, p. 211) but he did not, to the best of my
knowledge, develop this suggestion in his later works.

Nonetheless, there are tacit but obviously ethical
implications in the way in which the norms of autonomy,
personal integration, insight, and responsibility
are understood (James and Jongeward, 1971, pp. 263-74).
These norms permeate the therapeutic process, for they
provide a context within which the notion of "progress"
takes its meaning.

In a very simplified fashion, then, the view of
man we find in Transactional Analysis is as follows.
(1) The initial locus for the problem of evil (pathology) is the childhood environment; we are born
with a psychological neutral nature, which is shaped
in healthy or unhealthy ways by parental influences.
(2) Through the insights gained and decisions made
in the therapeutic process, we can neutralize internal conflicts and achieve substantial personality
integration.

177

III.

One way to look at the two views I have presented is to see them simply as appropriately different ways to understand different dimensions of our life, one the theological dimension, the other the psychodynamics of the human personality. One aims at salvation, the other at health. The fact that the two goals are not synonymous is shown by the fact that we find no conceptual problems in conceiving of an atheist who enjoys good mental health or of a deeply religious person who suffers from a psychosis. Likewise, we do not believe that a psychosis normally can be cured by religious practices alone. So it is plausible to argue that each approach addresses a different aspect of human life in an appropriately different fashion.

On at least one occasion Berne took this kind of position when he wrote that structural analysis in no ways tries to encroach into the "well-defined" areas of the philosopher, the theologian, and the lawyer; and "neither does it expect to be dragged into any of them against its will" (Berne, 1972, p. 326). The problem, however, is that the theoretical reach of each kind of understanding of man's psyche tends to extend into the domain of the other. The line between them is far from distinct, as we also shall see in the next two sections. Insofar as they both represent interpretations of the human condition, they often seem to be not merely different but competing and incompatible views. Moreover, when a pastoral counselor considers using structural analysis, he can hardly be expected to pretend his psychology and theology can remain in splendid isolation from each other.

Questions remain. For example, is aggressive and destructive behavior to be understood as pathologically dysfunctional behavior to be treated by psychotherapy? Or is it to be understood as sinful conduct, evidence of moral failure, calling for confession, repentance, and atonement? Or is it both? Our labels are crucial, for what behavior is <u>called</u> "determines which type of help the sufferer receives--medical, legal, social, pastoral" (Menninger, 1973, p. 93).

It is easy to see how, from the point of view of Christianity, humanistic psychotherapies such as

178

Transactional Analysis may seem to be attempts to interpret sin and sinfulness in purely naturalistic terms, and therefore represent a secularism of salvation, another form of Pelagianism, a renewal of the ancient Adamic rebellion of man trying again to be like God, now by trying to exorcise himself of his demons and transform himself apart from repentance and the redeeming and sanctifying power of God. If we have a conflicted nature and always will, Transactional Analysis (and any theory like it) also is impossibly utopian, for it tells us we can effectively work toward and achieve internal integration, and moreover do it by our own power, apart from the help of God.

Likewise, from the point of view of humanistic psychotherapeutic theory, Christianity, at least as I depicted it, can be seen as promoting pathology, first by teaching that it is unavoidable and then by making sure it is in fact unavoidable by commanding its adherents to be without sin, to measure themselves against a humanly unobtainable goal of perfection. "You, therefore, must be perfect as your heavenly Father is perfect" (Matt. 5:48).[2] If a child is told again and again that he has a sinful will which must be broken, he is bound to grow up with a "gamy" or "scripty" life plan. Christianty puts people in a totally no-win situation; it is no wonder, then, that so much pathology manifests itself in religious ways.

IV.

Perhaps, however, it is possible to reconcile a humanistic psychotherapy such as Transactional Analysis with Christianity. One such effort "to integrate a psychological system with a theological position: has been made by Muriel James (1973) a disciple of Berne and an ordained Congregational minister.

Dr. James' "integration" actually amounts to

---

[2]Several readers of this paper have told me that this quotation should not be understood literally but should be taken to mean something like "be fully what you are created to be." Nonetheless, this admonition often is understood literally by ordinary readers of the Bible, and even if the textual interpretation is incorrect, the point of the criticism is still clear.

a psychologizing of theology. By the expression, "psychologizing of theology," I mean that the naturalistic theory of man found in TA and its categories are used not merely to gain psychological insight into the social dynamics of the church but also to interpret and stand in judgment over theological doctrines.[3] Dr. James writes: All churches periodically evaluate their theology. . . . Transactional Analysis can be used both for evaluation and to initiate desired change" (p. 62). The desired changes, the goals which act as norms for a desirable theology are getting our transactions with others straightened out and achieving intimacy with others. Doing this, she writes, is "a redeeming experience that enables the church to be more effective" (p. 99).

TA theory gives James no alternative except to hold that any church which takes the position that people are sinners who need saving, is assuming either an "I'm not-OK, You're not-OK" or an "I'm OK, You're not-OK" position. Unfortunately, the first position must be characterized clinically as "schizoprhenic or schizoid," leading to depression and disintegration; and the second is "arrogant and clinically paranoid" and manifests itself in critical and blaming attitudes towards others, chronic advice giving, and even persecution (pp. 92-3). Both positions inevitably give rise to all sorts of pathological transactions with others, "games" such as "I'm Only Trying to Help You" and "Blemish." These "games," played from a moralistic Parental ego-state, are based upon and reinforce the view that people are sinners, in a "not-OK" position (pp. 114-6, 124-5).

The only mentally healthy position, James writes, is the "I'm (we're) OK, you're (they're) OK" position. Her implicit recommendation is that the traditional doctrine of original sin must be regarded as a psychologically unhealthy aberration. And, as we have seen, the inevitable result of deemphasizing the doctrine of original sin is to also de-emphasize the

---

[3]It also is possible to psychologize in a philosophic position or argument, if the latter is analyzed only in terms of the ego-state of the author, and the analysis or argument itself remains unexamined in terms of such philosophic canons as clarity, accuracy, and cogency.

traditional doctrines of redemption and grace.

James provides only one example of that type of psychological criticism which requires a radical reinterpretation of theological beliefs. It would be easy to multiply citations from other humanistic psychotherapists who explicitly denounce the traditional doctrine of original sin. To do so, however, would be only to repeat the point James already has made: there apparently are fundamental incompatibilities between humanistic psychology and traditional Christianity.

V.

Dr. James' psychologizing of theology is only one way of trying to integrate psychotherapy and theology. It also is possible to theologize psychotherapy, that is, to interpret and judge psychological categories, theories and methods on the basis of theological beliefs. Doing so, as we might expect, seems inevitably to mean a radical revision of psychotherapeutic theory and practice. Let me make some suggestions about how this kind of reconstruction _might_ proceed.

A Christian might begin by pointing out that, even in TA theory, it is perfectly appropriate for a person to feel "not-OK" when he finds himself in a non-OK situation, say, one involving the death of a loved one. Now a person finds himself in a not-OK situation as a sinner, and "the menaing of the 'good news'. . . is that, although unacceptable, I am accepted" (Tillich, 1963, p. 222). Therefore, there is nothing wrong or not OK with his seeing himself and others as _being_ not-OK (ontological sinfulness and theological guilt) nor with his _feeling_ not-OK (psychological guilt), and, because he now is accepted by God, as seeing himself (and others) is _also_ in an OK status with the right to feel OK about himself (and them).

If this view more accurately takes into account the complexitites of our human nature, it is right that we should always have a certain ambivalence about ourselves and others; and any more simplified view misrepresents reality and cannot provide a theoretical basis for such integration as we can hope to achieve in this life.

Just as the beginning point--the Christian view of

181

human nature--is radically different from the humanistic view, so also the end of Christian counseling
turns out to be radically different from the goals of
humanistic psychotherapy. In traditional Christianity
there is no such thing as an autonomous or self-
actualizing person or a fully functioning person. We
always are limited by the given structures of creature-
hood and discipleship. As a consequence, the very
notions of "responsibility" and "integrity" take on
very different meanings from those given them in psychotherapy.

From psychology, the Christian counsellor may
borrow empirically sound insights into the dynamics
of the human personality and of the interpersonal relationships; and he also may feel bound, both by his
Christian faith and by the dynamics of the counseling
situation, to accept unconditionally the person who
comes to him. But insofar as his counseling is
specifically Christian, he cannot deny his conviction
that sin is real, that guilt and shame can be legitimate, and that moral reformation cannot be adequately
understood merely as a natural process.

VI.

There is another way to integrate psychotherapy
and theology, which seems to dissolve, not merely resolve, many of the problems we have seen (Bouwsma,
1976).

According to W.J. Bouwsma, we cannot begin to
identify a specifically Christian conception of what
it is to be a healthy adult without first distinguishing between the authentic source of that conception
in Biblical Christianity and inauthentic sources which
he describes as cultural accretions to historical
Christianity, originating as far as classical antiquity.

It was classical rationalism, Bouwsma writes,
which introduced the dualistic picture of man as a
complex of body and soul, of desires and reason. It
was the same classical philosophy which analyzed the
human species in terms of an absolute, static goal of
"manhood" rather than in terms of the processes of
human development. "Manhood" was identified with the
rule of reason which had the function of subduing and
suppressing the "lower" passions. When incorporated

182

into historical Christianity, Bouwsma writes, this
fundamentally non-Christian concept led to the view that
the mature Christian is a person who, feeling guilt for
his persistent attraction to lower things, undertakes
a rigorous asceticism as the means to save his soul.

By contrast, Bouwsma writes, the normative Biblical conception of creation resists dichotomous contrasts
between child and adult and between desire and reason.
Because "man was created as a whole, indeed in God's
image, every aspect of man is good and worthy of development, for 'God saw all that he had made, and it
was very good' (Gen. 1:31)" (p. 82). Moreover, because creation took place in time, full adulthood is
not an end but an ongoing process, a capacity for
indefinite growth (since the goal of full conformity
to the manhood of Christ is unattainable in this life).
The source of all particular sins consists, like the
original fall, in people seeking to become "like gods"
by rejecting change and refusing to admit the need for
further growth.

Insofar as Christian theology remains tied to
merely human and cultural absolutes, Bouwsma implies,
it can easily impede the best genuine interests of
Christians. And insofar as we recover the normative
Christian conception of human adulthood, we will see
there is no necessary conflict between the psychological
category of dysfunctionality and the Christian conception of sinfulness; both refer to the person caught in
immaturity. Both Christianity and psychotherapy see
the solution in terms of the recovery of the capacity
for and the resumption of growth, requiring the rein-
tegration of the dichotomized self, the acceptance and
cultivation of the qualities of the child as part of
adulthood, and the replacement of guilt-ridden re-
pressive behavior by freedom and spontaneity.

On this view of sin and sancification, psychotherapy offers a complementary, not a competitive, view
of adulthood, but one which needs supplementing only
by the Christian emphasis on man's dependence on God,
and the roles of faith and grace as conditions for
genuine growth, autonomy, and freedom.

If there is a single major problem here, it concerns the rightness of Bouwsma's claim that creation-
theology rather than redemption-theology most

authentically reflects Christianity. Bouwsma admits
that creation-theology "has rarely been dominant in the
history of Christianity" (p. 82). Obviously it is not
within my area of expertise as a philosopher to try to
decide what is and what is not the authentic Christian
view.

VII.

In this paper I have not tried to decide what is
the 'right' view of man, and I also have avoided difficult questions about relations between psychological,
moral, and religious/theological concepts. As important as such questions are, an adequate discussion
would require a book, not an article.

My purpose has been to set out, as clearly as
possible, the separate anthropologies operative in
naturalistic psychotherapy and in traditional Christianity and to show the influence of each anthropology.
I also have tried to show that any integration of
psychotherapy with Christianity depends heavily on
how notions like "sin" and "psychological health" are
understood.

The problems are particularly relevant to the
practice of psychotherapists who also are traditional
Christians. During the 1970's most of the historic
tensions between traditional Christianity and psychotherapy seemed to dissipate almost completely, and
questions such as those raised by Karl Menninger (1973)
were quietly brushed aside and ignored. This irenicism
now seems destined to show some severe strains. Studies
indicate that we now are in the middle of a return to
traditional values, and insofar as this means a re-
emphasis of "redemption-theology," it is inevitable
that old tensions between humanism and Christianity
will gain new attention.

Christian counselors and particularly pastoral
counselors who have adopted the methodology of
structural analysis such as that found in Transactional
Analysis find themselves living a life of conceptual
schizophrenia, living in two very different worlds
with incompatible commitments. Their life may tend to
fall apart just at the point where they are trying to
help others achieve integrity. I have used the word

184

'may', because a widespread acceptance of "creation-process theology" or something similar (e.g. Hoffman, 1979) could signal the beginning of a new age of Christian humanism, in which contemporary psychological insights are integrated with a deeply Christian conception of human nature and human destiny.[4]

---

[4]I am deeply grateful to Thomas O. Buford, C.J. Hammet, Edwin M. Hadley, Jr., Leander E. Keck, Eugene T. Long, and Kenneth W. Taber for their criticisms of earlier drafts of this paper. Each disagreed with some part or other of the paper, and none should be held responsible for the opinions I have expressed. I particularly want to thank William F. Rogers, III, my student, who, on the basis of his own pastoral counseling, helped me through the several drafts.

THE THERAPEUTIC INGREDIENTS OF RELIGIOUS AND

POLITICAL PHILOSOPHIES

Edith Weisskopf-Joelson

When I immigrated to the United States in 1939
as a refugee from Hitler, one of my most interesting
new experiences pertained to the realm of religion.
In the old country I was raised without much religious
education. Most of my relatives, my friends, and I
were agnostics or atheists. (I was Jewish by descent
rather than by faith.) Therefore, I was most interested and bewildered about the strong religious
experiences described to me by some of my students
and acquaintances in the United States. One of my
most striking discoveries were the Campus Crusaders
for Christ. Here were young men and women who had
been deeply unhappy, disinterested in their studies,
in their future careers, in their future marriages.
Some were well on the way towards becoming alcoholics
or drug addicts. "Then," they tended to say, "I became a Christian." What did they mean? They must
have been Christians since birth as I had been Jewish
since birth. But they viewed the situation differently! They were Gentiles since birth, but not Christians. Most often they spoke of one day in their
adolescence when they prayed for Christ to come into
their lives which they had done many times before, but
on that day it happened. It was an experience of
absolute certainty: Christ had not been in their
lives at 3:00 p.m., but at 3:05 p.m., He was there.
The experience was blissful, led to continuing happiness, to the conviction of being saved and to the obligation to lead others to salvation. Witnessing of this
kind may seem trite to those listeners who have heard
it many times before, but it was new, baffling, interesting and thought provoking to me.

These powerful religious conversions reminded me
of equally powerful "conversions" which I have observed
between March and September 1938 in Austria occupied
by Hitler. For example, a friend of mine related that
he had felt lost and desperate before he went to his
first meeting of the Nazi Party. After he had left
the meeting he wrote into his diary: "Now my life has
meaning!"

Much later I had a similar experience of my own.
The New Women's Liberation Movement fundamentally
altered my self-concept and my relationships to others
in a radiantly positive direction.

Experiences of this kind led me to the following
questions: How does it come about that religious and
political philosophies can endow a human life with
happiness, meaning, and fulfillment? What are the ingredients of religious and political movements which
have the power to heal?

I approached these problems with a double purpose.
On the one hand I considered the possibility of obtaining some "hard-nosed" data on questions such as these:
"What kind of healing ingredients do different religious and politic faiths contain?" or "Do people
of different personality structures, of different
sex, of different age benefit from different faiths?"

On the other hand I wanted to find a faith for
myself. This chapter deals more with the latter than
with the former attempt; at this point I have not
counted, tabulated and statistically analyzed the
healing ingredients of faith; instead I have attempted
to experience them, to feel them, to empathize with
the believer. Therefore, I will describe and discuss
the various healing aspects of faith with the intention
of letting the readers participate in this empathy--
to help them experience, by using especially moving or
expressive quotes from religious and political writings,
what support or nourishment by faith feels like. Most
of the quotes are taken from the religious faith and
the political movement with which I am experiencially
most familiar, namely from Roman Catholicism, the
overwhelming majority faith in Austria, and from
National Socialism, which I have directly experienced
as a potential victim and vicariously experienced as
an observer of party members.

My materials where the "bibles" of religious and
political faiths, such as the Holy Bible, the Torah,
the Koran, the Upanishades, Hitler's Mein Kampf; in-
terviews, diaries and autobiographies of believers;
participation in worship services and in one Nazi mass
meeting; visits to the communes or temples of a
variety of cults such as the Hare Krishnas, the

Theosophists, etc. I also used transcripts from therapy sessions of believers; however, the latter are neither quoted nor discussed for reasons of confidentiality.

Occasionally, I shall refer to philosophical systems other than religious and political ones.

The remaining part of the chapter describes and discusses the healing ingredients which I found.

A. Support

A philosophy offers support by relating the believer to entities which he perceives as being greater than himself. From these entities he may receive 1. consonance, 2. strength, 3. love, 4. annihilation, and 5. embedment into eternity.

1. Support through Consonance

It is a comfort to be surrounded by people who share our views. Thus, fulfillment springs not only from the creed of a philosophy but also from the fact that it is believed by others. Rokeach and others (Byrne & Wong, 1962; Rokeach, 1960; Rokeach & Mezei, 1966) report that communality of opinion is a more important determinant of mutual attraction than "race". (Triandis, 1961, reports contrary results.)

The members of a religious congregation are linked to each other by a common view of the human condition. The contemporary decline of religious faith has given rise to numerous substitutes for congregations which are often based on more specific communalities than the entire human condition. In groups such as Alcoholics Anonymous people find in others what they find in themselves. The same is true for other self-help organizations, most of which could be subsumed under the label "Neurotics Anonymous". It is an interesting observation that patients, who are treated by the same therapist, or by therapists of the same school, tend to associate with each other in what they view as social cliques but what are actually quasi-religious communities.

The mere knowledge that there are people who see the world as we do--though we might never have met

189

these people--may give us Support by endowing us with
invisible friends. It is a paradox that even the
very view that there are no ties between us and others
(Camus, 1955) may establish such ties if it is a
shared view.

2. Support through Strength

Here the believer is endowed with strength and
power by becoming a part of a powerful entity.

Nationalistic world views, for example, tend to
offer the believer this kind of Support. Many
nationalists feel strong, important, and glamorous
because they are a part of a nation which they perceive as strong, important- and glamorous. A leader
might make young followers feel that they are a part
of their nation by words such as these:

> Whatever we may create today, whatever we do - we
> shall have to pass away. But in you our country
> will live on, and when nothing will be left of
> us, you will hold in your fists the flag which
> we raised up from the void. And you must stand
> firmly on the soil of your earth, you must be
> strong so that this flay never slips from your
> hands, and then, after you, let generation after
> generation come: you can ask of these that they
> become as you had been (source unknown).

It is noteworthy that in the above illustration
the supporter demands strength in addition to giving
it. The concomitance of strength-endowing Support
and the demand for strength may not be coincidental.

It is conceivable that in contemporary religious or
political faiths which are palatable to Western individuals, strength-endowing Support tends to be
camouflaged by the demand for strength based on individual effort rather than on Support. This might
be the case because people with even moderately individualistic orientations would not be able to feel
strong and powerful if they were told explicitly that
they are weak and powerless as individuals, and were
to borrow from a supporting source of strength. The
admonition "Ask not what your country can do for you.
Ask what you can do for your country" (Kennedy, 1961,
p. 278), may serve as an extreme illustration of this

attitude, for here strength-endowment is being demoted in favor of demand for strength.

We would expect to find examples of strength-
endowing Support without the demand for strength in
the Judeo-Christian faiths. An example (Stein, 1967):

> I know myself held[by God] , and in this I have
> peace and security--not the self-assured
> security of a man who stands in his own strength
> on firm ground, but the sweet and blissful se-
> curity of the child which is carried by a strong
> arm, considered objectively a no less reasonable
> security. Or would the child be "reasonable"
> who lived in constant fear that its mother might
> drop it? Hence in my being I meet another, which
> is not mine, but is support and ground of my un-
> supported and groundless being. (p. 247)

Strength-endowing support can stand alone without
the demand for strength in the Judeo-Christian ethic
because Judeo-Christianity was originated in a con-
siderably less individualistic setting than the present Western world. One could hypothesize that contemporary, and especially American interpretations of
Judeo-Christianity would tend to deemphasize the manifest expression of Strength-endowing Support. The
nothingness of the human being alone, without the
support of God and Jesus Christ, would tend to receive
less stress than in the Bible. Rabbi Liebman's (1946)
attitude is a drastic manifestation of this predicted
trend. Under the heading "A new God idea for America"
he writes:

> I am making the prophecy that it will be
> from the democratic experience of our
> century that mankind will first learn its
> true dignity as independent and necessary
> partners of God....
> . . . .
> One of the greatest troubles is that in our
> religion we have continued to picture our
> relationships to God in terms of the help-
> less, poverty-stricken, powerless motifs in
> European culture. Now, a religion that will
> emphasize man's nothingness and God's
> omnipotence; that calls upon us to deny our
> own powers and to glorify His--that religion

191

may have fitted the needs of many Europeans,
but will not satisfy the growing self-
confident character of America....(pp. 159-
160)

A hyper-democratic relationship to God is also
portrayed in Fiddler on the Roof, where Tevye chas-
tises the Lord. Likewise, "One great Hasidic rabbi,
Levi-Yitzhak of Berditchev, once warned God, 'If you
refuse to answer our prayers, I shall refuse to go on
saying them." It was Levi-Yitzhak, too, who one day
addressed God in exasperation: "Master of the Universe, how many years do we know each other? How
many decades? So please permit me to wonder: Is this
any way to rule your world?" (Time, April 1, 1972,
p. 58).

The reluctance of the contemporary American man
to accept help from God is reflected in the following
joke: A farmer is exceedingly successful in restoring a very delapidated farm. His minister comments,
"With Our Lord and you in charge this farm has developed beautifully." Whereupon the farmer replies, "You
should have seen it when Our Lord was in charge alone!"

3.   Support through Nurturance

Every step which the child undertakes in his development toward maturity brings about the necessity
to forego more infantile gratifications. Thus, developmental progress is often accompanied by considerable nostalgia. Growing up means losing the privilege
of entertaining sweet, dependent, protected relationships which are based on self-centered receiving rather
than on a give-and-take basis. For example, the satisfaction of passive, irresponsible sucking at the
mother's breast has to be given up, first for the sake
of more active, less convenient cup-and-spoon feeding,
which lacks the intimate physical contact with the
mother and burdens the child with heavy responsibility,
and much later for the strenuous and inconvenient
activity of making a living. Intellectual growth, too,
means renouncement of the satisfaction of dependency
needs. Learning to read may mean to a child not being
read to; learning to think may mean not being thought
for; learning to get oriented in the environment may
mean not being guided and protected (Weisskopf, 1951).

No wonder that many people yearn to reestablish a childlike state of bliss where they can receive love, care, nurturance, and protection, needs which receive little satisfaction in American society. In a society where independence is a high value, dependency needs can be satisfied, for example, by neurotic avenues such as illness, by semineurotic avenues such as acquiring an excessive number of college degrees to postpone maturity, or by highly acceptable avenues such as satisfying children's dependency needs and, then, getting vicarious enjoyment from their satisfaction. But the royal road to dependency are religious faiths. "In a sermon which probably shocked his Victorian congregation, Hopkins, the Jesuit poet, compared the Church to a cow with full udders, patiently waiting for the world to come and be fed" (Scharper, 1959, p. 49).

Goethe's (1882, b) poem to follow may serve as another illustration of Nurturing Support.

Wanderer's Night-Song

Thou that from the heavens art,
Every pain and sorrow stillest,
And the doubly wretched heart
Doubly with refreshment fillest,
I am weary with contending!
Why this rapture and unrest?
Peace descending
Come, ah, come into my breast! (p. 53)

The French Catholic writer Peguy (1945) sees God as satisfying man's dependency needs in a very un-American manner. In his book God speaks, he writes:

The man who is in my hand like the staff
   in the traveller's hand,
That man is agreeable to me, says God.
The man who rests on my arm like the suckling
   child who laughs
And sees the world in his mother's and his
   nurse's eyes,
And sees it nowhere else, and looks for it
   nowhere else,
That one is agreeable to me, says God.
(pp. 34-35)

The most powerful examples of the loving support offered by Christianity can be found among the passionate statements of Christian Saints about their relationship to God: "Oh, night that guided me, oh, night more lovely than the dawn, oh, night that joined Beloved with lover, Lover transformed in the Beloved!" (St. John of the Cross).

Assuming that Catholicism offers nurturant Support to a higher degree than Protestantism, we might hypothesize that one of the etiological factors of Anti-Catholic attitudes in the United States is the rejection of dependency needs in the American culture. This rejection tends to make Americans perceive people who are not inhibited in fulfilling such needs as threatening. Such threats might be based on unconscious envy, and on the somewhat realistic fear that the possibility of fulfilling dependency needs within the Catholic faith may make repression of such needs more difficult for the non-Catholic. Thus, the psychological relationship of the non-Catholic to the Catholic in the United States might be compared to the relationship of the former alcoholic to the drinker: seeing another person drink may make it hard to control drinking for someone with overwhelming longing for alcohol.[1]

4. Support through Annihilation

Schweitzer (1939) characterized this kind of Support as follows: "The Indian idea of the divine is, that it is pure, spiritual essence. It is the ocean into which man, tired of swimming, wishes to sink" (p. 38).

The Eastern mind yearns for the Support of complete merging with the supporter: The supported one ceases to exist and he becomes an inseparable and indistinguishable part of nature by being dissolved into particles of soil, water, or living matter.

---

[1]In this context it is of interest to note that the Protestant Jaroslav Pelikan (1959) discusses many motives for conversion to Catholicism, without mentioning as a possible motive the desire to receive more nuturant, protective, personal, and warm support than Protestantism can offer.

With their individualistic attitudes, Occidentals find it difficult to perceive such annihilation as Support. They are unable to see Support where there is no one to be supported. In contrast, Orientals experience the faith in resurrection and immortality which is so comforting to the Christian as an un-bearable burden! Such faith precludes any hope of merging with the absolute for all eternity (Guirdham, 1959).

But the supreme happiness is the achievement of Oneness, in being joined to God and to all things visible and invisible. In orthodox Christianity even the saved soul is still separate. We will sit on the right hand of God in the Glory of the Father. Heaven is full of majesty and glory but there will, even in our glory, be separation from the Father, the Son, and the Angels. (p. 60)

An oriental proverb says the first 35 years of a man's life should be dedicated to the task of severing himself from the dust from which he originated; and the second part of life to the task of becoming dust again and, thus, of returning to the source of his origin. Gradual disintegration into dust during the afternoon of life is not a threatening notion to the Eastern mind. I shall leave it to the reader's imagi-nation to picture the response to this metaphor of American men slightly above the age of 35; or even the response of the American public to making it a corner-stone of a basic philosophy of gerontology!

Especially in Catholicism with its strong in-fluence from Oriental religions one can find many sub-tle transitions between Support through Nurturance and Support through Annihilation. Perhaps the difference is one of degree rather than one of kind, since love implies some loss of identity "even though the death which ensues from it is very little death and its implications of Oneness very fleeting and often illusory" (Guirdham, 1959, p. 149).

5. Support through Time-expansion

This kind of support is based on strengthening the believer's emotional relationship to time periods transcending the personal life span by creation of

195

metaphysical ties, or by glorification of empirical
ties, with the past and the future; thus, it soothes
the pain of finitude.[2]

---

[2]Time-annihilating philosophies are closely related to time-expanding ones; but views tend to dull
the pain caused by the passage of time (Guirdham,
1959).

Those devoted to the mystical aspects of the
Eastern religions and who practice their special
postural and meditative techniques are enabled
to achieve a state of being in which considerations of time and space are annihilated. In contrast, there is a powerful emphasis on time in the
Christian faith, and emphasis which Orientals tend
to view as torturous and antithetical to healing.
It is the special boast of Christianity that of
all religions it has the most historical justification. (It is a little doubtful whether this
is true. The facts of Mahomet's career are at
least as well known and verifiable as those of
Christ.) Certainly, however, the historical
facts relating to the origin and spread of
Christianity are far better defined than is the
case with Buddhism and Hinduism. But it may well
be that Christianity has erred greatly in seeking to locate God in history. That God became
incarnate nearly two thousand years ago may be
comforting to the Christian afflicted with these
historical and legalistic preoccupations with
which he chooses to prove the truth of his
religion at the cost of losing understanding of
its nature. It does, nevertheless, limit the
extent of God's sphere of operations. The gift
of the Holy Spirit at Pentecost, at a fixed date
after the Crucifixion, embodies a concept of
religion which is completely at variance with
that of a universal spirit infusing all things
from a beginning which was never a beginning to
an end which will never end. In contrast, the
essentials of the Christian faith are that Christ
was the Son of God incarnate in man, that He was
born of a virgin in a village at a certain
date. . . . (pp. 75-77) (Italics mine.)

(1) Metaphysical ties to the future and to the past.

    a. Future

       Faith in immortality is the purest example, taken from Christianity, of Time-expanding Support based on metaphysical ties to the future.

    b. Past

       Metaphysical ties to the past are established, for example, by the Catholic Holy Communion as described by Scharper (1959):

> ...I am... aware that God is within me and I try to respond to that fact. In me, at this moment all history meets and whatever I know of reality engulfs me--I have received Christ, "born of the Father before all ages," who "under Pilate was crucified" yet who "lives and eeigns forever." I feel that the ancient myths meet in me and are clarified. I have been with Beowulf beneath the sea and gone with Orpheus beneath the earth. (p. 47)

(2) Glorified empirical ties to the future and to the past.

    a. Heredity

       Biologically heredity creates empirical ties to future and past, but these objective ties may not be potent enough to defeat death -- the dreadful enemy -- unless they are endowed with radiance and splendor through ideological emphasis.

The sense of eternity bestowed on us by contemplation of our ancestors and our offspring may be aggrandized to a fortissimo as follows:

> In you lives the heritage of millions of ancestors, the bloodstream of the entire race. Behind your two parents stay four grandparents, eight great-grand-parents and so forth. Each earlier generation doubles the number of your ancestors. In the twenty-fifth generation there are already

more than thirty-three million of them; twenty-
five generations--that takes about 600 years. Of
all these sixteen million men, of all these
sixteen million women you are a part, a wisp, a
feeling, a thought. They all live on in your
body, in your blood, immortal to this day.
Sixteen million men and sixteen million women have
woven your fabric, have bequeathed to you their
strength or their weakness. The whole race of
you are your ancestors, as they are all ours.
Thus, too, is the history of your people your own
history. Our common blood and our common history
make us brothers. In this great community your
blood, your soul, lives on. It lives in your
deeds and your words, in your thought and dreams
and will once be in your children and theirs.
In you pulsates the blood of the singers and
poets of the folksongs and the heroic epics, of
the masters who built the domes, of the painters
and woodcarvers of immortal works of art....
(Source unknown).

    b. Cultural transmission

     Every man is eternal insofar as he makes a
lasting imprint on his environment. As Faust (Geothe,
J.W., 1882, a) says: "The traces cannot, of mine
earthly being, in aeons perish, -- they are there! --"
(p. 295).

B. <u>Strengthening of our ties to reality by
rapproachement of private and official interpretations of human existence</u>.

    Many of us feel elated about the child who
said "the emperor does not have any clothes." We
would be less elated if we focused on the moments,
hours, days, weeks, months, and years which preceded
this statement. During that time the child had to
face the painful experience of knowing that the
shared, official interpretation of the scene was
diametrically opposed to his or her private interpretation. Much of the grief which we experience stems
from such discrepancies. The feces which seem to
smell so sweet and look so handsome to the two-year-old
are "really" disgusting. The long-haired music leaves

the eight-year-old cold, while the egghead parents listen with rapture which the child is expected to share. The first kiss seems a little disgusting and a little ridiculous to the twelve-year-old while the world resounds of the glory of young love.

And as our two-year-olds grow up to be eight, twelve, seventeen, twenty-five and forty, and to approach death, and as the discrepancies add up, they learn to keep their own views to themselves in silent loneliness. And then it happens. First a whisper, then many audible voices, then a chorus in unison: "The emperor does not have any clothes." A philosophy has arisen. Now there is harmony between the private and public image of life; separation is overcome; union is established. "When we adopt a philosophy we discover, as it were, the I in a theory . . . . the outer and the inner world become integrated by such adoption, since the philosophy of life partakes in outer as well as in inner reality" (Weisskopf-Joelson, 1968, p. 369).

Discrepancies between private and official views are most painful if official interpretations of life are happy ones and private interpretations are saddening and gray. Then even frightening and pessimistic views may become balm against alienation. Perhaps it is easier to be united in sadness than to be alone in joy.

How this healing ingredient can be expected to affect people of different psychological and demographic characteristics is a problem which is accessible to empirical investigation.

A specific question pertaining to this general problem is the effect, on the reader, of existential literature which portrays the "hollow" aspect of life. To what degree does such literature evoke feelings of connectedness, and to what extent does it evoke feelings of despair? Is there any interaction between psychological and sociological characteristics of the reader, and the degree to which he or she can achieve union by pessimistic views of life?

C. Strengthening of our ties to reality by rapproachement of primary and secondary thought processes through myths, symbols, and rituals.

World views can enhance mental health in still
another way: they often counteract our alienation from
reality by achieving a union between primary and
secondary thinking.

A brief explanation of the distinction between
primary and secondary thought processes is in order.
The normal adult member of a complex society engages
in primary thought processes mainly in dreams. During
waking life primary processes may enter into thoughts
or determine actions by merging with secondary ones.
Conversely, young children and psychotics tend to
think predominantly along primary channels.

Primary thoughts are altogether determined by
our unconscious impulses. Their validity is not submitted to any reality testing and their functioning is
not subject to the rules of Aristotelian logic. A
normal adult may dream of a person who is his father
and at the same time his son (condensation). The
notion that such a person could exist is absurd within
the reference-frame of external reality; yet, it is
psychologically meaningful if the dreamer's personal
relationship to his father and to his son have much
in common; if, within the symbolic vocabulary of his
unconscious, the meanings of "father" and "son" are
the same. In contrast, secondary thought processes are
directed toward the assessment of external reality.
They are validated by the criterion of accurate
prediction of specific classes of phenomena.

The contemporary Occidental is culturally biased
so as to underestimate the importance of primary
thought processes, and to emphasize the importance of
secondary ones. This bias is justified when it applies
to the scientific prediction of certain phenomena,
but it is fallacious with regard to the prediction of
others. The primary thought process by which "father"
and "son" are merged into one concept lacks efficiency
for many pruposes. It would be impractical for the
purpose of formulating laws regarding human behavior
as a function of age, or of changing cultural conditions. It would make the formulation of some legal
principles utterly impossible, and would throw complete confusion into any attempts of census-taking.
But when it comes to explaining certain irrational
actions of the dreamer who merged his father with his
son, insight into primary thinking might be much more

important than insight into secondary thinking. For example, the dreamer's primary thoughts might explain why he relates to his son in an inappropriate manner which would, however, be an entirely appropriate way of relating to his father.

For our present purpose one specific aspect of the distinction between primary and secondary processes is of utmost importance. Sometimes during the socialization process the individual has to renounce the predominance of primary thought processes in favor of secondary ones in order to survive in the physical and social surroundings. This renunciation represents perhaps one of the most painful and difficult tasks of growing up. It is the most sacrificial experience of separation in human life; it is a separation from a part of ourselves, from our most authentic and spontaneous wishes, fantasies, and images which are not in accordance with objective reality. For the first time, we are confronted by the "implacable otherness" of the world which has become an object, to be assessed critically, analytically and without subjective bias.

Such a traumatic separation leaves with us a longing, usually unconscious, to recapture what we have lost. The psychotic succeeds in doing so, but this success is based on forfeiting contact with reality. Nevertheless, recapturing the lost inner world is a desire that presses for fulfillment. If it remains unfulfilled, life seems meaningless and hollow. Ideally, such fulfillment should be attained in a manner which is compatible with the maintenance of contact with external reality, for example, through shared symbolic rituals and myths.

The Catholic myth that the wine of the Eucharist Sacrament is the blood of Christ, and that the ressurection is being relived at every Holy Mass, is absurd when evaluated on the basis of secondary thought processes; but it is consonant with the thought processes of the unconscious (Jung, 1958, pp. 247-298). A myth of this kind could conceivably be someone's dream even though the dreamer may never have been exposed to the Catholic creed. Just like dreams and other primary thoughts, the mystic ritual of the Mass is characterized by visual images, by identification of the symbol with the symbolized object, and by lack of distinction between similarity and identity.

Thus, symbolic rituals make primary thoughts a part of external reality. Now the world is no longer an altogether alien object. Instead, it includes our intimate fantasies; fantasies which are so incompatible with external reality that they could never have entered it by any other vehicle than the one of myths, symbols, and rituals.

Through the vehicle of myths and symbols the believer is again a part of the world, and the world is a part of the believer. The abyss of separation has been bridged and the feeling of belongingness and unity has been reestablished.

Knowledge increases our control over nature, but myth has no real purpose, as some might say; it is "merely" an illusion which "for thousands of years has wrung from man the greatest spiritual effort, the loveliest works of art, and the profoundest devotion, the most heroic self-sacrifice, and the most exciting service" (Juny, 1958, p. 250).

The last two healing ingredients (pp. 16-21) are closely related to each other. In one case the healing effect is based on rapproachement between two conscious interpretations of life, one private and one official, in the other case on rapproachement between unconscious primary thought processes and conscious secondary ones. In both cases healing takes place through union of the subjective and the objective, of our inner lives and our external world. Elsewhere (Weisskopf-Joelson, 1968) I have used the term "halfway house" for enterprises which bring about such a union. Just as a half-way house (in the original meaning of the word) fulfills the subjective needs of its vulnerable residents, and simultaneously permits them to meet the demands of society, a metaphorical half-way house counteracts alienation by fusing our inner lives with our outer world.

D. Values

A system of values is a part of most, if not all, philosophies of life. It is a set of beliefs that certain modes of behaving, thinking, feeling, or perceiving are most desirable than others; value systems convey to the believer which causes are worth striving for, or fighting against. Values present us with a relief of our existence, showing as mountains what is important, as valleys what should be demoted to the realm of irrelevance.

It would be an endless task to discuss the rationales for the hypothesis that values may be among the healing ingredients of philosophies. I shall forego this task and limit myself to discussing, of the many possible rationales, only one which is frequently overlooked in spite of its far-reaching implications.

First I need to digress. The threat of failing to materialize all the potentialities of our personal lives forms an inherent part of human existence. This failure cannot be avoided even by the person who makes the best possible use of all possibilities for self-realization: every choice, be it the choice of a vocation, of a personal relationship, of an ideological belief, of a social responsibility, or of any other commitment, implies the rejection of other possible choices. Saying "Yes" to one possibility means saying "No" to an infinite number of others. Endowing one small part of the unborn future with life means killing an infinite number of other parts, and accepting the pain and guilt of the "Either-Or" predicament (Kierkegaard, 1944). Describing his search for a purpose to live by, the protagonist of Wheelis' (1960) novel The Seeker says, "Henceforth I would be aware ... of the necessity and fatality of choice--each choice being the death of what I would have become had I chosen otherwise, and being another step toward death for the person I was becoming through such choices" (p. 26). Value systems may mitigate this pain and guilt by reducing the number of possible choices. Metaphorically speaking, value-oriented ideologies take the burden of the believer's guilt upon their own shoulders; instead of leaving the responsibility of murdering the unborn future to humans, they take it upon themselves by supplying a map of the narrow road on which to travel.

For a deeply devout Christian such as the Trappist monk who wrote the following passage, the burdens of choice-making and of wasted opportunities have lost much of their weight; they rest in the hands of God (Merton, 1955).

Our Father in Heaven has called us each one to the place in which He can best satisfy His

203

infinite desire to do us good. My vocation is the one I love, because it is the one God has willed for me. If I had any evidence that He willed something else for me, I would turn to that on the instant. Meanwhile, my vocation is at once my will and His. I did not enter it blindly. He chose it for me when His inscrutable knowledge of my choice moved me to choose it for myself. I know this well enough when I reflect on the days when no choice could be made. I was unable to choose until His time had come. Since the choice has been made, there have been no signs in favor of changing it, and the presumption is that there will be no change. That does not mean there <u>cannot</u> be a change. (p. 138)

The above illustration suggests that the relief offered by value systems through reducing the number of possible choices might be outweighed by the predicament of the initial choice of a value system, and the exclusion of other value systems. The believer, like the person who borrows from a loan company, exchanges all small debts for a single, comprehensive and all-embracing one.

Even the Western world in the twentiety century which is somewhat opposed to the direct dissemination of values, seems to find indirect ways of disseminating values. An especially interesting indirection of this kind is the tendency of depth psychology to replace the concept "Value" by the concept "unconscious impulse". The modern way of saying "you should" is to say "you have the unconscious impulse to do so," an impulse which has to be brought into awareness (Weisskopf, 1952). If I were a modern prophet I would disguise myself as a psychotherapist and would declare my Ten Commandments not as commandments but as unconscious potentialities of which we have to become aware. I would not say "Thou shalt love thy neighbor as thyself," but, instead, "Thou has an unconscious desire to love thy neighbor, and this desire must be brought into consciousness." This is the contemporary way of speaking and thinking about values.

The modern Western hesitation with regard to direct dissemination of values can be illustrated by the following fragments from the psychotherapy of

204

a young, male patient (De Grazia, 1952). Here the therapist disseminates a psychoanalytically oriented world view. But instead of openly advocating sex as something desirable he beats around the bush, and finally induces the patient to say, "Sex is natural; sex is within me."

PATIENT: Perhaps I am scared of a girl because I am terrified that my sexual feelings might run away with me, and I might not act rationally.

THERAPIST: What might you do?

PATIENT: I might love her too much.

THERAPIST: What would that lead to:

PATIENT: My desire would be to put my arms around her, and tell her I love her. But I was scared.

THERAPIST: Does that seem so terrifying?

PATIENT: Well, I might lose control and go too far.

THERAPIST: How far might you go?

PATIENT: Well, I might have sexual intercourse with her:
That would be going too far.

THERAPIST: Would it?

PATIENT: Well, perhaps not as far as sexual intercourse. If that is the devil, perhaps he is quite a harmless devil. Perhaps the sooner I went to the devil the better.

THERAPIST: If that is all there is to it, why is there all this scare?

PATIENT: Apparently all this time I have been afraid of being possessed by my own nature. The thing I want more than anything else is to lead a normal, life. Since coming to you I have

> understood that this fear of being sold
> to the devil is nothing more or less
> than fear of my own nature on the one
> hand, and on the other hand a pre-
> ference for it, which I have thought
> was a preference for the devil. The
> whole amazing thing has become quite
> plain to me. It is amazing how the
> obsession left me last night after that
> talk with you. (pp. 100-102, Italics
> mine)

If a "metatherapist" were to reflect, in a Rogerian fashion, the feelings underlying the therapist's
comments, he might remark: "You are trying to say,
'Why the hell don't you screw her!'" But the therapist
does not say so. Instead, the patient has to find
his values within himself.

The fact that many therapists tend to wash their
hands of any responsibility with regard to the dissemination of values is also shown in the following comment
made by Frankl (Standal & Corsini, 1959) about a
therapist who says to his promiscuous female patient,
"I forbid you to sleep with another man." Frankl
comments: "There is no question whatever of authori-
tative interference in the case under consideration.
The therapist simply verbalized what the patient already subconsciously knew. Is it not, ultimately,
the task of psychotherapy to make unconscious knowledge available, so the patient can manage it, and
thereby become more aware of it?" (p. 33). Again,
Frankl puts values inside the patient, instead of
admitting the obvious fact that the therapist has
disseminated values from the outside.

E. Acceptance of Unavoidable Suffering

We have many means at our disposal which
enable us to avoid unhappiness and suffering. Within
limits we have learned to control diseases, combat
starvation, and the like. But suffering certainly
has not been entirely eliminated from human existence.
The aspect of philosophies which I wish to discuss
does not attempt to remove the external sources of
suffering. Instead, it attempts to convert the believer's rejection of unalterable suffering to

acceptance and surrender. For example, "homo patients" (Frankl, 1950), the suffering being, may be viewed as more Christ-like and, thus closer to God than others, not in spite, but because of unalterable suffering.

The feeling of warm intimacy and loving pride towards the inevitable pain in one's life is in drastic contrast to the attitude prevailing in the United States, where the incurable sufferer is given very little opportunity to be proud of unavoidable suffering, to consider it a road to ennoblement rather than to maladjustment. Our martyrs elicit psychiatric attention rather than religious devotion. In addition to being unhappy, we are unhappy about being un-happy (Weisskopf-Joelson, 1955). Wolfenstein (1951) calls this American attitude towards suffering "fun morality": it is ethically desirable to be happy and to have fun. She illustrates this by saying that an old-fashioned girl felt guilty on a date when she had a great deal of fun; a modern girl feels guilty when she does not have fun.

Such notions may be responsible for the fact that the complaints of many psychiatric patients are pre-dicaments which should not, or cannot be eliminated from their lives. The real disease is sometimes not the complaints which motivated patients to seek help, but the fact that they view these complaints as enemies and not as friends.

Thus, viewpoints which convey the message "it is all right to suffer, to be anxious, to be depressed," may be balm for persons who do not only suffer, but who, in addition, suffer because they suffer.

For psychotherapists--Frankl (1963) being an ex-ception--convey such "pathophylic" philosophies of life. Psychotherapy often "fosters the belief that [all] unhappiness is an illness, a product of local and temporary conflicts, and that it can be cured" (Wheelis, 1960, p. 46).

F. Ambiguity

Ambiguity is the amount of leeway left to the believer regarding the interpretation of an ideology. This healing ingredient, in contrast to the previous ones, is independent of the concrete content of philosophies; instead, it refers to the manner in which the content is presented to, and received by, the believer.

In some ways Protestantism is more ambiguous than Catholicism. For example, Jesus, Mary, and the saints are presented to the Catholic by paintings and statues which give a definite picture of their physical characteristics; this is the case to a much lesser degree for the Protestant.

The healing power of Ambiguity might be explained as follows: a somewhat ambiguous philosophy gives us the opportunity to shape our creeds in accordance with our own inner lives, and, thus, to experience them individually rather than collectively.

Different personalities might be expected to respond in different manners to differences in ambiguity. Some people love to see their favorite novels on the screen; others respond to such concreteness with depression, because they have been deprived of the possibility to shape their fictitious friends according to their own fantasy. Similar feelings may be aroused when they have the misfortune of meeting their idols, such as psychotherapists, film stars, football players, and the like, in concrete, social situations. It often seems that "holy, sweet, redeeming uncertainty" is "our supreme consolation" (Unamuno).[3]

G. Meaning

Frankl (1962) has stressed that a meaning, a purpose, a goal in life is the most important need of human beings.

Political philosophies tend to set goals, such as the communist state or the Third Reich. But according to Frankl the meaning of a human life is unique for each individual, and common political goals are often experienced as coercion. Moreover, political dreams for the future often prove grossly dissappointing and/or grossly immoral when they become reality, as the above two examples show.

---

[3]The exact source of this quotation could not be located.

Also many religious philosophies point towards common goals, such as salvation, but for many believers they may also point to the unique goals and purposes of their individual lives. This is the case if the believer feels that God has endowed him or her with a unique personality and with the duty to use this personality for specific purposes. This feeling of having a mission in life can be the source of enormous energy, endurance, persistence, conviction and ecstacy.

To find our uniqueness and the meanings of our lives we must be still, we must empty ourselves, we must wait, we must avoid the temptation to escape, to drown our emptiness in an ocean of constant activity and distraction. Jesus went into the desert to find the meaning of his life.

To find meaning in the future we must be able to endure the abysmal suffering of living without meaning for days, weeks, months, and sometimes for years, of leading lives without meaning, lives without goals, lives which seem to come from nowhere and lead to nowhere. And then, someday, we shall feel the gentle touch of the great enigma which some of us call God.

BIBLIOGRAPHY

BIBLIOGRAPHY

Agel, J. The Radical Therapist. New York: Ballantine Books, 1971.

Allport, G., Becoming: Basic Consideration for a Philosophy of Personality. New Haven, Conn., Yale University Press, 1955.

_____. The Individual and His Religion. New York, Macmillan, 1950.

Aristotle. Nicomachean Ethics c. 340 B.C. . Trans. M. Ostwald. Indianapolis, Ind.: The Bobbs-Merrill Company, Inc., 1962.

Ayer, A.J., ed. Logical Positivism. New York: Free Press, 1959.

Bakan, D. Sigmund Freud and the Jewish Mystical Tradition. Princeton: Van Nostrand, 1958.

Beck, Carlton E. Philosophical Foundations of Guidance. Englewood Cliffs, N.J.: Prentice-Hall, Inc. 1963.

Berenda, C., "Is Clinical Psychology a Science?" American Psychologist, 1957.

Berger, P. "Toward a Socialogical Understanding of Psychoanalysis," in Facing Up to Modernity, Berger, P., ed. New York: Basic Books, 1977, Chap. 2, pp. 23-34.

Bergin, A. "Psychotherapy and Religious Values," Journal of Consulting and Clinical Psychology, 1980, 48, 95-105.

Berne, E. What Do You Say After You Say Hello? New York: Grove Press, 1972.

_____. Transactional Analysis in Psychotherapy. New York: Grove Press, 1961.

Bloch, Donald A.: cited in Buhler, 1962, p. 180.

Boring, E.G. A History of Experimental Psychology (2nd ed.). New York: Appleton-Century-Crofts, 1950.

213

Bouwsma, W.J. "Christian Adulthood." Daedalus, 1976, 2.

Breuer, J. & Freud, S. On the Psychical Mechanism of Mysterical Phenomena: Preliminary Communication. In J. Strachey (Ed.), The Standard Edition of the Complete Psychological Works of Sigmund Freud (Vol. II). London: Hogarth, 1955.

_____. Theoretical Selection, Section III. In J. Strachey (Ed.), The Standard Edition of the Complete Psychological Works of Sigmund Freud (Vol. II). London: Hogarth, 1955.

Brown, P.H. Radical Psychology. New York: Harper & Row, 1973.

Buber, M. Hasidism and Modern Man. New York: Horizon Press, 1958.

_____. I and Thou. New York, Scribner's, 1968.

Bugental, James F.T., ed. Challenges of Humanistic Psychology. New York: McGraw-Hill, Inc., 1967.

Bugental, James F.T. The Search for Authenticity. New York: Holt, Rinehart and Winston, Inc., 1965.

Bühler, Charlotte. "Human Life as a Whole as a Central Subject of Humanistic Psychology." In Challenges of Humanistic Psychology, ed., J.F.T. Bugental. New York: McGraw-Hill, Inc., 1967.

_____. "Humnaistic Psychology as a Personal Experience." Journal of Humanistic Psychology, 1979, 19, 5-22.

Bühler, Charlotte and Allen, Melanie. Introduction to Humanistic Psychology. Monterey, Calif.: Brooks/Cole Publishing Co., 1972.

Bühler, Charlotte. Values in Psychotherapy. New York: The Free Press of Glencoe, 1962, p. 16.

Burckhardt, Titus (Stoddart, W., trans.) <u>Alchemy</u>.
    London: Stuart & Watkins Lts., 1967.

Byrne, D. & Wong, T.J. "Racial Prejudice, Inter-
    personal Attraction, and Assumed Dis-
    similarity of Attitudes." <u>Journal of
    Abnormal and Social Psychology</u>, 1962, <u>65</u>,
    246-253.

Camus, A. <u>The Myth of Sisyphus and Other Essays</u>.
    New York: A.A. Knopf, 1955.

Clark, W.H., <u>The Psychology of Religion</u>. New York,
    Macmillan, 1958.

Clement, P., "Getting Religion," <u>American Psycho-
    logical Association Monitor</u>, June, 1978.

Curran, C.A., "Counseling, Psychotherapy, and the
    Unified Person," <u>Journal of Religion and
    Health</u>, 1963.

DeGrazia, S. <u>Errors of Psychotherapy</u>. Garden City,
    N.Y.: Doubleday & Company, 1952.

Ellis, A. <u>Humanistic Psychotherapy: The Rational-
    Emotive Approach</u>. New York: Julian Press,
    Inc., 1973.

Epictetus, <u>The Enchiridion</u>. Indianapolis: Bobbs-
    Merrill Co., 1955.

Faulkner, W., "Nobel Prize Address." Reprinted in
    O.W. Vickery, eds., <u>William Faulkner:
    Three Decades of Criticism</u>, East Lansing,
    Michigan, Michigan State University Press,
    1960.

Frank, Jerome D. <u>Persuasion and Healing</u>. Baltimore:
    The Johns Hopkins Press, 1961, p. 10.

_____. <u>Persuasion and Healing</u>. Baltimore:
    Johns Hopkins Press, 1973.

Frankl, Victor. From Death Camp to Existentialism. Boston: Beacon Press, 1959.

_____. Homo Patients: Versuch Einer Pathodizee. Vienna: Deuticke, 1950.

_____. Man's Search For Meaning. Boston: Beacon Press, 1962.

_____. Man's Search For Meaning: An Introduction to Logotherapy. New York: Washington Square Press, Inc., 1969.

_____. "Self-transcendence as a Human phenomenon." In A.S. Sutich and Miles A. Vich, eds., Readings in Humanistic Psychology. New York, The Free Press, 1969.

_____. "The Concept of Man in Logotherapy." Journal of Existentialism, 6, 53, 1965.

_____. The Doctor and the Soul. New York: Alfred Knopf, 1955.

Freud, S. "A Case of Successful Treatment by Hypnotism." In J. Strachey (Ed.), The Standard Edition of the Complete Psychological Works of Sigmund Freud (Vol. I). London: Hogarth, 1966. (a)

_____. A New Series of Introductory Lectures in Psychoanalysis. New York: Norton, 1933.

_____. "Contributions to a Discussion on Masturbation." In J. Strachey (Ed.), The Standard Edition of the Complete Psychological Works of Sigmund Freud (Vol. II). London: Hogarth, 1958.

_____. "Lines of Advance in Psychoanalytic Therapy," Standard Edition, 1919, Vol. 17.

_____. "On Narcissism: An Introduction." In J. Strachey (Ed.), The Standard Edition of the Complete Psychological Works of Sigmund Freud (Vol. XIV). London: Hogarth, 1957.

_____. "Project For a Scientific Psychology. "
In J. Strachey (Ed.), _The Standard Edition_
of the Complete Psychological Works of
Sigmund Freud (Vol. I). London: Hogarth,
1966. (b)

_____. "Some General Remarks on Hysterical
Attacks." In J. Strachey (Ed.), _The Stan-_
dard Edition of the Complete Psychological
Works of Sigmund Freud (Vol. IX). London:
Hogarth, 1959.

_____. "The Aetiology of Hysteria." In J.
Strachey (Ed.), _The Standard Edition of the_
Complete Psychological Works of Sigmund
Freud (Vol. III). London: Hogarth, 1962
(b)

_____. "The Neuro-Psychoses of Defense." In J.
Strachey (Ed.), _The Standard Edition of the_
Complete Psychological Works of Sigmund
Freud (Vol. III). London: Hogarth, 1962.
(a)

_____. _The Origins of Psycho-Analysis, Letters_
to Wilhelm Fliess, Drafts and Notes:
_1887-1902_. New York: Basic Books, 1954.

_____. "The Psychopathology of Everyday Life." In
J. Strachey (Ed.), _The Standard Edition_
of the Complete Psychological Works of
Sigmund Freud (Vol. VI). London: Hogarth,
1960.

_____. _The Standard Edition of the Complete_
Psychological Works of Sigmund Freud (Vol.
_II)_. London: Hogarth, 1955.

Fromm, Erich. _Escape from Freedom_. New York: Holt,
Rinehart and Winston, 1941.

Ginsburg, Sol W., and Herma, J.L.: cited in Buhler,
1962, pp. 10-11.

Glover, Edward, _The Technique of Psychoanalysis_. New
York: International Universities Press,
1958.

217

Goethe, J.W. _Faust: A Tragedy_. (Taylor, B., Trans.).
       Boston: Houghton, Mifflin, and Co.,
       1882. (a)

_____. "Wanderer's Night-Song." In _The Poems of_
       Goethe. (Longfellow, W., Trans.). New
       York: Crowell & Co., 1882.

Goldstein, Kurt. _Human Nature in the Light of Psycho-_
       pathology. Cambridge: Harvard University
       Press, 1940.

_____. _The Organism_. New York: American Book
       Company, 1939.

Guirdham, A. _Christ and Freud: A study of religious_
       experience and observance. London: Allen
       & Unwin, 1959.

Havens, J., _Psychology and Religion_. Princeton, New
       Jersey, D. Van Nostrand Company, Inc.,
       1968.

Hixon, L. _Coming Home: The Experience of Enlighten-_
       ment in Sacred Traditions. Garden City:
       Anchor Books, 1978.

Hobbs, N. "Sources of Gain in Psychotherapy." _Ameri-_
       can Psychologist, 1962, _17_, 741-747.

Hoffman, J.C. _Ethical Confrontation in Counseling_.
       Chicago: The University of Chicago Press,
       1979.

Horney, Karen. _Neurosis and Human Growth: The_
       Struggle Toward Self-realization. New
       York: Norton, 1950.

Jahoda, Marie. _Current Concepts of Positive Mental_
       Health. New York: Basic Books, 1958.

James, M. _Born to Love_. Reading, Mass.: Addison-
       Wesley Publishing Co., 1971.

James, M. and Jongeward, D. _Born to Win_. Reading
       Mass.: Addison-Wesley Publishing Co.,
       1971.

Jones, E. The Life and Work of Sigmund Freud: The
          Formative Years and Great Discoveries (Vol.
          1). New York: Basic Books, 1953.

Jung, C.G. Civilization in Transition. In H. Read,
          M. Fordham, & G. Adler (Eds.), The
          Collected Works of C.G. Jung (Vol. 10).
          Bollingen Series XX.10. New York:
          Pantheon, 1964.

_____. "Freud and Psychoanalysis." In H. Read, M.
          Fordham, & G. Adler (Eds.), The Collected
          Works of C.G. Jung (Vol. 4).
          Bollingen Series XX.4. New York: Pantheon,
          1961.

_____. The Collected Works of C.G. Jung. Vol II.
          New York: Pantheon Books, 1958.

Kant, I. Religion Within the Limits of Reason Alone
          [1973]. Trans. Greene and Hudson. New
          York: Harper and Row, Pub., 1960.

Kennedy, J.F. Inaugural Address of Jan. 20, 1961.
          In Meyersohn, M. (Ed.). Memorable Quo-
          tations of John F. Kennedy. New York:
          Crowell Co., 1965.

Kierkegaard, S.A. Either-or: A Fragment of Life.
          Vol. I., (Swenson, D.F., & Swenson, L.M.,
          Trans.). Princeton, N.J.: Princeton
          University Press, 1944.

Krasner, L. "The Operant Approach in Behavior Therapy,"
          in Bergin, A. and Garfield, S. (Eds.)
          Handbook of Psychotherapy and Behavior
          Change. New York: Wiley, 1971. 612-652.

Lewin, K. A Dynamic Theory of Personality: Selected
          Papers. New York: McGraw-Hill, 1935.

Liebman, J.L. Peace of Mind. New York: Simon &
          Schuster, 1946.

Livermore, Joseph M., Malmquist, Carl P., and Meehl,
          Paul E.: "On the Justifications for Civil
          Commitment." University of Pennsylvania
          Law Review. 117, 1968.

219

Macklin, Ruth: "Mental Health and Mental Illness: Some Problems of Definition and Concept Formation." Philosophy of Science, 1972; and "The Medical Model in Psychoanalysis and Psychotherapy." Compr. Psychiatry, 1973.

_____. "Norm and Law in the Theory of Action." Inquiry. 11: 400-409, 1968.

Mahoney, M.J. Cognition and Behavior Modification. Cambridge, Mass.: Ballinger Publishing CO., 1974.

Margolis, Joseph: Psychotharapy and Morality. New York: Random House, 1966.

Maslow, Abraham. "Comments on Dr. Frankl's Paper." In A.J. Sutich and M.A. Vich (Eds.), Readings in Humanistic Psychology. New York: The Free Press, 1969.

_____. Eupsychian Management: A Journal. Homewood, Illinois, Richard D. Irwin, 1965.

_____. Motivation and Personality. New York: Harper, 1954.

_____. Religions, Values and Peak Experiences. Columbus, Ohio, Ohio State University Press, 1964.

_____. Toward a Psychology of Being. Princeton New York: Van Nostrand, 1962.

May, Rollo. (Ed.). Existence. New York: Basic Books, 1961. (b)

_____. Existential Psychology. New York: Random House, 1961 (a)

_____. "Intentionality: The Heart of Human Will," Journal of Humnaistic Psychology, 1964.

_____. Love and Will. New York: Norton Press, 1969.

McGuire, W. (Ed.), The Freud/Jung Letters. Princeton,
        N.J.: Princeton University Press, 1974.

Menninger, K. Whatever Became of Sin? New York:
        Hawthorn Books, Inc., 1973.

Merton, T. No Man is an Island. New York: Harcourt,
        Brace & Co., 1955.

Monte, C. Beneath the Mask. New York: Praeger, 1977.

Morris, Joe E. "Humanistic Psychology and Religion:
        Steps Toward Reconciliation." Journal of
        Religion and Health, 19, 92-102.

_____. "Kierkegaard's Concept of Subjectivity and
        Implications for Humanistic Psychology."
        Journal of Humanistic Psychology, 1979.

Nagel, E. The Structure of Science: Problems in the
        Logic of Scientific Explanation. New York:
        Harcourt, Brace, & World, 1961.

Niebuhr, R. The Nature and Destiny of Man, Vol. I.
        Human Nature. New York: Charles Scribner's
        Sons, 1964.

Patterson, C.M.: cited in Buhler, 1962, p. 17.

Peguy, C. "Abandonment." In God Speaks: Religious
        Poetry. (Green, J., Trans.). Pantheon
        Books, 1945.

Pelikan, J.J. The Riddle of Roman Catholicism. New
        York: Abingdon Press, 1959.

Polanyi, M., Personal Knowledge. Chicago, University
        of Chicago Press, 1958.

Popper, K.R. The Logic of Scientific Discovery.
        London: Hutchinson, 1958.

Progoff, I., Jungs Psychology and Its Social Meaning.
        New York, Gove Press, 1953.

Rieff, P. Freud: The Mind of the Moralist. New
        York: The Viking Press, 1959.

Riordan, K. "Gurdjieff" in Transpersonal Psycho-
        logies. Tart, C., ed. New York: Harper
        & Row, 1975, chap. 7, pp. 281-326.

Roberts, D.E. Psychotherapy and a Christian View of
        Man. New York: Charles Scribner's Sons,
        1950.

Rogers, Carl. "A Theory of Therapy, Personality and
        Interpersonal Relationships, as Developed
        in the Client-Centered Framework." In S.
        Koch (Ed.), Psychology: A Study of a
        Science. 3 vols. New York: McGraw-Hill,
        Inc., 1959.

_____. Client-Centered Psychotherapy. Boston:
        Houghton-Mifflin, 1951.

_____. Client-Centered Therapy, Its Current
        Practice, Implications, and Theory. Boston:
        Houghton Mifflin, 1951.

_____. On Becoming a Person. Boston: Houghton-
        Mifflin Co., 1961.

_____. "Persons or Science." In Frank T. Severin
        (Ed.), Humanistic Viewpoints in Psychology.
        New York: McGraw-Hill, 1965.

Rokeach, M. & Mezei, L. "Race and Shared Belief as
        Facotrs in Social Choice." Science, 1966,
        151, 167-172.

_____. The Open and Closed Mind. New York:
        Basic Books, 1960.

Royce, J., "Metaphoric Knowledge and Humanistic Psy-
        chology." In J.F.T. Bugental, ed.,
        Challenges of Humanistic Psychology. New
        York, McGraw-Hill, 1967.

_____. "Psychology, Existentialism, and Re-
        ligion," Journal of General Psychology,
        1962.

Rychlak, J.F. "Carl Gustav Jung as Dialectician and
Teleologist." In G.S. Saayman & R.K.
Papadopoulos (Eds.), Contemporary Approaches
to Jungian Thought. London and Johannes-
burg: Ad. Donker, in press.

_____. A Philosophy of Science For Personality
Theory. Boston: Houghton Mifflin, 1968.

_____. The Pychology of Rigorous Humanism.
New York: Wiley-Interscience, 1977.

Sandler, J., Holder, A., and Dare, C. "Basic Psycho-
analytic Concepts: VII. The Negative
Therapeutic Reaction." British Journal of
Psychiatry, 1970, 117, 431-436.

Scharper, P. "What a Modern Catholic Believes."
Harper's Magazine, 1959, 218, 40-49.

Schur, M. Freud: Living and Dying. New York: In-
Ternational Universities Press, Inc., 1972.

Schweitzer, A. Christianity and the Religions of The
World. (Powers, J., Trans.). New York:
Holt, 1939.

Severin, Frank T. (Ed). Humanistic Viewpoints in
Psychology. New York: McGraw-Hill, Inc.,
1965.

Shapiro, A. "Placebo Effects in Medicine, Psychotherapy, & Psychoanalysis," in Bergin, A.
& Garfield, S. (Eds.) Handbook of Psychotherapy and Behavior Change. New York:
Wiley, 1971. 439-743.

Sollod, R. "Carl Rogers and the Origins of Client-
Centered Therapy," Professional Psychology,
1978, 93-104.

_____. "Ethical Issues in the Relation of Re-
ligion to Psychotherapy." Presentation to
the 86th annual A.P.A. convention, Toronto,
1978a.

Snygg, D., & Combs, A.W. Individual Behavior: A New Frame of Reference For Psychology. New York: Harper & Brothers, 1949.

Standal, S. & Crosini, R. (Eds.). Critical Incidents in Psychotherapy. Englewood Cliffs, N.J.: Prentice-Hall, 1959.

Stein, E. Cited in Stein, W.J. & Edith Stein, Twenty-Five Years Later. Spirtual Life, 1967, 3, 244-251.

Sullivan, R.J. Morality and the Good Life: A Commentary on Aristotle's "Nicomachean Ethics." Memphis, Tenn.: Memphis State University Press, 1977.

_____. "The Kantian Critique of Aristotle's Moral Philosophy: An Appraisal." The Review of Metaphysics, XXVII, 1 (Sept. 1974).

Sutich, A.J., and Vich, M.A. (Eds.) Readings in Humanistic Psychology. New York: The Free Press, 1969.

Szasz, T.S. The Myth of Mental Illness. New York: Hoeber-Harper, 1961. Ausubel, D.P.: "Personality Disorder is Disease," in Scheff, T.J. (Ed.): Mental Illness and Social Processes. New York: Harper and Row, 1967.

Tart, C. "Some Assumptions of Orthodox, Western Psychology," in Transpersonal Psychologies, Tart, C., ed. New York: Harper & Row, 1975, chap. 2 pp. 59-112.

Tillich, P., "Psychoanalysis, Existentialism and Theology," Pastoral Psychology, 1959, 9, 9-17.

_____. The Courage to Be. New Haven, Connecticut: Yale University Press, 1952.

_____. The Courage to Be. New Haven, Conn., Yale University Press, 1957.

_____. Systematic Theology. Chicago, University of Chicago Press, 1951, 1.

_____. Systematic Theology, Vol. 3. Chicago: The University of Chicago Press, 1963.

Toulmin, S. "From Logical Analysis to Conceptual History," in P. Achinstein & S.F. Barker (Eds.) The Legacy of Logical Positivism. Baltimore: John Hopkins University Press, 1969, 525-537.

Triandis, H.C. A Note on Rokeach's Theory of Prejudice. Journal of Abnoral and Social Psychology, 1961, 62, 184-186.

Van Kaam, Adrian. "Assumptions in Psychology." In Frank T. Severin (Ed.), Humanistic Viewpoints in Psychology. New York: McGraw-Hill, Inc., 1965.

Vaughn, R.P., "Existentialism in Counseling: The Religious View," Personal and Guidance Journal, 1965, February.

Vitz, P. "A Christian Critique of Academic Secular Personality Theory." Presentation to the 88th annual A.P.A. convention, Montreal, 1980.

_____. Psychology as Religion: The Cult of Self-Worship. Grand Rapids: Eerdmans, 1977.

Wachtel, P. Psychoanalysis and Behavior Therapy: Toward an Integration. New York: Basic Books, 1977.

Watson, G. "Areas of Agreement in Psychotherapy." American Journal of Orthopsychiatry, 1940, 4, 698-710.

Websters New World Dictionary. New York, World Publishing Company, 1960.

Weisskopf, E.A. Intellectual Malfunctioning and Personality. Journal of Abnormal and Social Psychology, 1951, 46, 410-423.

Weisskopf-Joelson, E. "Meaning as an Integrating Factor." In Buhler, C. & Massarik, F. The course of human life. New York: Springer, 1968.

_____. "Some Suggestions Concerning Weltanschauung and Psychotherapy." Journal of Abnormal and Social Psychology, 1953, 48, 601-604.

_____. "Some Comments on a Viennese School of Psychiatry." Journal of Abnormal and Social Psychology, 1955, 51, 701-703.

Weisskopf, W.A. "Theoretical Role of Psychodynamics." Ethics, 1952, 62, 184-190.

Welkowitz, J. Personal Communication. New York University, June, 1978.

Wertheimer, Michael. "Humanistic Psychology and the Humane But Tough-minded Psychologist." American Psychologist.

Wheelis, Allen: cited in Buhler, 1962, p. 13.

_____. The Seeker: A Psychoanalyst's Search For His Own Life's Meaning. New York: Random House, 1960.

White, R.W. Personal Communication. Harvard University, October, 1978.

Wittels, F. Sigmund Freud: His Personality, His Teaching, and His School. New York: Dodd, Mead, 1924.

Wolberg, L.R.: cited in Buhler, 1962, p. 173.

Wolfenstein, M. "The Emergence of Fun Morality." Journal of Social Issues, 1951, 7, 15-25.

Wolff, Werner: cited in Buhler, 1962, pp. 11-12.

Woitzky, D. and Silverman, L. "Controversies in Psychoanalysis: Can They be Resolved?" unpublished manuscript. New York University, 1980.

Wolpe, J. "Cognitive Behavior and its Roles in Psy-
          chotherapy: An Integrative Account,"
          in Psychotherapy Process: Current Issues
          and Future Directions. Mahoney, M.J. ed.
          New York: Plenum Press, 1980, chap. 7,
          pp. 185-202.